How To Be A Hypnotherapist

BY LORRAINE GLEESON

'ENLIGHTENED, AMUSING AND
EXTREMELY ACCESSIBLE'
William Broom

Copyright © 2013 Lorraine Gleeson
All rights reserved.
Edited by Lesley Hussell
ISBN: 148128603X
ISBN-13: 9781481286039
CreateSpace Independent Publishing Platform
North Charleston, South Carolina

Table of Contents

Table of Contents	iii
About the Author	xv
What the experts say	xvii
Introduction	xix
Chapter One	**1**
Introduction to Hypnosis	1
What is hypnosis?	1
My golden rules	3
The induction	4
The keys to an effective induction	7
Guidelines for using your induction script	7
A word about scripts ...	8
Noises	9
Music	9
Recognising the trance state / gauging depth	10
Awakening	11
Practising hypnotherapy	13
Advice on recording software and equipment	13

Recommended microphone	14
Free recording software	14
Other recording software	14
Recording tips	14
Note – insurance	14

Chapter Two — 19
The Holistic Theory of Man — 19

The two-part theory of man – the medical profession's viewpoint	19
The holistic theory of man – the hypnotherapist's viewpoint	20
The conscious and the subconscious mind	21
The origin of client problems	27
Life influences and the creation of unique individuals	28
The importance of establishing causes	29

Chapter Three — 33
Suggestibility — 33
The Finger Test — 33
Suggestion — 33
The language of hypnosis — 33
Arm assurance — 33

Purpose of the finger test	33
What to do if the fingers do not part	35

Why the finger test works	36
Suggestion – the language of hypnosis	38
Direct suggestion	38
Indirect suggestion	39
The four rules governing suggestion	40
The language of hypnosis	42
Terminology to avoid	43
The arm assurance procedure	44

Chapter Four   51
Deepening The Hypnotic State &
IMR – Ideo-Motor Response   51

Recognising the trance state / gauging depth	51
When to use deepeners	52
IMR – Ideo Motor Response	53
What is IMR?	53
Why do we use IMR?	53
Explaining IMR to your client before hypnosis	53
Positioning the client's hands	54
The stages of the process are broken here:	56
Creating new behaviours/alternative choices – NLP technique	58
The choice of finger and their meanings	60
Trouble shooting –	60
Reasons why a finger does not respond:	61
Too deep in hypnosis	61
Just not playing	61

Chapter Five — 69
Regression — 69
- Preparation for the second session — 69
- Pre-induction conversation — 70
- Regression — 70
- Regression outline — 71
- Protection — 73
- Tips for successful regression — 73
- What to do once you get a response — 74
- When regression 'doesn't work' — 75
- Distance feelings — 77
- Gestalt technique — 78
- Inner child / higher self — 80
- Concluding the session — 82

Chapter Six — 91
Questioning and Maintaining Rapport — 91
Avoiding non-leading questions — 91
- Open questions, closed questions and when to use them — 92
- Leading and non-leading questions — 94
- The danger of leading a client during hypnosis — 94
- Tips for questioning during regression — 96
- Establishing the cause — 96
- The next step – reprogramming — 97

Chapter Seven — 99
Neuro Linguistic Programming (NLP) — 99
- NLP – what is it? — 99
- Who started it? — 100
- Understanding the principles of NLP – visual, auditory and kinaesthetic — 100
- Working with NLP – effective client communication — 101
- Picking up non-verbal signals — 102
- Anchors — 103
- NLP techniques — 104
- Pain control — 104
- Treating headaches following hypnosis — 105
- Note on treating bereavement — 105
- Rewriting history — 105
- Creating new behaviours — 107
- Timeline — 108
- How it works — 108
- Action questions — 109
- How to help a friend (and yourself) by Michael Colgrass — 109
- NLP glossary — 110

Chapter Eight — 113
The Basic Formula — 113
Reprogramming therapy — 113
- The basic formula — 114

First visit – hypnotherapy	114
Next visit – facilitating change	114
Subsequent appointment/s – reprogramming	115
Personal view: just me and my client	116
Visualisation	116
Creating visualisations and reprogramming	117
Confidence reprogramming	117

Chapter Nine 125
More Inductions 125
Writing scripts 125
Self-hypnosis 125
Hypnosis for childbirth 125

More inductions	125
Rapid inductions	126
The hand drop instant induction	126
Mental confusion or analytical inductions	128
Writing scripts	131
Self-hypnosis	135
Before teaching self-hypnosis	136
Childbirth	136

Chapter Ten 139
Smoking 139

Aversion therapy	140
Focusing on benefits	140

Preparation	**140**
Questions	**141**
Weight	**141**
How many sessions – and what to charge?	**142**

Chapter Eleven 147
Weight Problems 147
1. Thin people have weight problems too	147
2. Diets do not work	147
3. How thin people think	148
4. Listening to your body, the benefits and changes	149
Building a therapy	150

Chapter Twelve 161
Fears and Phobias 161
Driving test nerves 161
Improving performance 161
Levels of fear	162
Fear and the body's chemical reactions	163
Top ten most commonly reported phobias in the uk	165
Common treatments	166
Drugs	166
Systematic desensitisation	166
Flooding	166
Treating fears with hypnotherapy	166

Hypnosis and desensitisation	167
'Taking control' technique	167
Driving test nerves	168
Improving performance	168
Summary	170

Chapter Thirteen — 179
Habits and Addictions — 179
More on behaviours — 179

Learned behaviour	179
Classical conditioning – Pavlov	180
Operant conditioning – Skinner	180
Cognitive conditioning	180
Learned helplessness	181
Repetition and reinforcement	181
Subconscious learning	181
Purposes of learning – conscious purposes	182
Purposes of learning – subconscious purposes	182
Tips for treating habits	182
Is the cause relevant?	182
Quitting a habit can leave a vacuum	183
Addictions	183
Physiological dependency	183
Psychological dependency	183
Treatment of addictions	183

Chapter Fourteen — 189
Working with Children — 189
- Hypnosis and children – the law — 189
- Is treatment of the child appropriate? — 189
- Working with children – the method — 190
- Conclusion — 191

Chapter Fifteen — 193
Neurobiology — 193
- **Neurobiology and hypnosis** — 193
- **Structure of the nervous system** — 194
- **Neurons** — 194
- **Multiple Sclerosis and hypnotherapy** — 196
- **The brain and CNS** — 197
- **The peripheral nervous system** — 198
- **Neuroplasticity** — 199
- **The brain and memory** — 199
- **Effects of hypnosis on the brain** — 200
- **Can we see what effect hypnosis has on the brain?** — 200
- **Hypnotherapists – beware** — 201
- **The relaxed brain and the active brain** — 203
- **Drugs** — 204

Chapter Sixteen — 209
Psychophysiological Disorders — 209
Medical classifications — 209

Causes of illness	209
What can hypnotherapy change?	210
Definition: a psychophysiological illness is 'a physical illness that has psychological causes.'	210
How can the mind create an illness?	211
The mechanics of the mind's influence	211
Muscle control, blood flow and pressure	212
Imbalance of the autonomic nervous system	212
Eating behaviour	212
Cell manufacture and regeneration	213
Healing	213
Energy field	213
Warning	213
Treating psychophysiological disorders	213
Medical classifications	219
Stress	219
Frustration	219
Conflict	219
Reactions to frustration	220
Aggression	220
Defence mechanisms	220
1. Denial	220
2. Repression	220
3. Rationalisation	221
4. Projection	221

5. Reaction formation	221
6. Intellectualisation	221
7. Displacement	221
Abnormal behaviour	221
Classifying abnormal behaviour	222
1. Neuroses	222
2. Psychoses	222
3. Personality disorders	223
Methods of treatment	223
Drugs	223
Counselling and group therapy	224
Electroconvulsive therapy (ECT)	224

Chapter Seventeen — 225
Setting Up in Business — 225

Qualifications and professional support	225
General hypnotherapy register (GHR)	226
Benefits	226
Membership of the Hampshire School of Hypnotherapy (HSH)	227
How can you describe your profession?	227
Insurance	227
Setting up your office/therapy room	228
Professional conduct	228
Client confidential records	229
National Occupational Standards	229
Accounts and taxation requirements	230

Marketing	**230**
Advertising standards	**231**

Appendix 233
My own experience of regression – never assume! 233
    Demands   239
    Needs   239

About the Author

Lorraine Gleeson had hypnotherapy in 2001 and it changed her life.

She trained as a hypnotherapist in 2004 with the Institute of Natural Therapies and is still very proud of the diploma she received. She set up practice in The Magick Bean, the coffee shop in Southsea on the south coast that she ran with her friend Steph Lyons. They had a little room in the back of the shop they fondly called Room 101. Customers kept dropping in to talk to Lorraine about their problems, so she eventually started charging for her help.

The INT was a great starting point but for a more practical course Lorraine went to Scarborough to train with Wilf Proudfoot at his school The Proudfoot School of Clinical Hypnosis and Psychotherapy. She received three diplomas in Clinical Hypnosis, Hypnotherapy and Neuro-Linguistic Programming (NLP).

Working with clients is one of the most rewarding things Lorraine has done and as she received more and more referrals, she found herself perfecting the techniques she had learned, blending them together to make them her own.

In 2007 she started to train hypnotherapists under the INT. Sharing her knowledge and watching other people become hypnotherapists was a fantastic experience, but Lorraine wanted to go one step further and train her own way, teaching people the techniques and formulas she knew first hand would work.

The Magick Bean was sold in 2009. Through the breakfast business networking group 4N, Lorraine learned from a lot of free advice and was inspired to start working from the Technopole Centre in Portsmouth, Hampshire. She wrote her own training course – the Hampshire School of Hypnotherapy manual – based on her personal experience as a hypnotherapist and with the help of a very patient Jan Paige.

Lorraine's confidence grew as she found that she could help more and more people. Having read Roy Hunter's book Inner Conflict, she flew the celebrated US hypnotherapist over to the UK in 2009 to teach Parts Therapy. She found Roy's client-centred approach so inspiring that in 2011 she flew him back again so that she could qualify to teach Parts Therapy.

Hampshire School of Hypnotherapy continues to grow, and all that Lorraine teaches is based on her own experience. It is what makes her approach so fresh.

Lorraine's passion for hypnotherapy is unbounded. Her success is down to her enthusiasm, her great sense of humour and the fact that she is not judgemental: she believes people can be whatever they want to be.

What the experts say

There are hundreds of books on hypnotherapy on the shelves and most of them should stay there! This book will appeal to both the novice just starting out and the experienced therapist wishing to up their game. Well written, easy to read, it should be in the collection of every hypnotherapist. It is already in mine!

John Maclean
Creator of the Hypno-Band System

Lorraine Gleeson has produced a work of unquestionable enlightenment within a theatre of human activity that has long been the subject of both myth and misunderstanding. She has fashioned a book that is by turn amusing, witty and, by shunning the use of technical jargon, extremely accessible. Although controversial in places in so far as not all practising hypnotherapists would necessarily agree with her underpinning philosophy of human nature and the way in which she consequently prefers to deliver her therapy, this book nonetheless provides a most comprehensive overview of what it actually entails – and feels like – to be a hypnotherapist.

With admirable generosity of spirit, the author liberally salts the text with personal anecdotes, all of which add subtle flavouring to a subject that, in some hands, might otherwise have turned into a somewhat dry and academic dish. Lorraine has an infectious enthusiasm for her chosen profession and this permeates every page.

I would recommend this book to anyone who may be interested in becoming a hypnotherapist as a most useful preliminary to undertaking the practical training required to realise that ambition. It will, at the very least, provide the reader with the necessary insight required to help decide whether the fascinating field of hypnotherapy is right for them, or not.

William Broom
Executive Advisor and Registrar
The General Hypnotherapy Standards Council and General Hypnotherapy Register

Introduction

Why have you bought this book – or why are you standing in the bookshop reading it? Because you want to learn hypnosis. Maybe you have experienced hypnosis before, perhaps being treated by a hypnotherapist or seeing a celebrity hypnotist perform.

How did you feel? What did you like? Think about this as you continue reading and begin to picture yourself as a hypnotherapist treating your own clients. This book, used in conjunction with a practical training course, will teach you how to facilitate lots of different techniques so you can become a therapist in your own right, incorporating a wide range of skills including scripts, regression, gestalt, self-hypnosis and Neuro-Linguistic Programming (NLP). You will be able to set up practice and feel confident you have the knowledge and skills to help your clients with many things, from weight loss or smoking to anxiety, fears and phobias.

This book on hypnotherapy is different, because my approach is different. On the first day of training I say to every group: "Do not believe anything I tell you or anything you read." There's usually silence! But you really do need to find out for yourself. I want my trainees to become therapists in their own right, not a carbon copy of me. As a hypnotherapist, you will need to have a lot of techniques in your toolbox so that you can be flexible and totally client centred. This is so important. If one technique fails with a client, you will be able to try something else. You need to work on your own initiative, act on your own feelings and trust what you think.

With this in mind, this book will teach you a selection of techniques and a very simple formula to follow. You will have a structure but also the creativity to be adaptable. I want you to think outside the box and try things – to really make a difference and help your clients be the best they can possibly be.

How to be a Hypnotherapist includes lots of practical advice, case studies, scripts, comments from some of my previous trainees (called 'Personal view'), fascinating facts and questions to help you test your knowledge as you go along.

You want to be a hypnotherapist – enjoy it!

Chapter One

Introduction to Hypnosis

Induction

Awakening

Practical Preparations

What is hypnosis?

Hypnosis is a very natural state. If you imagine consciousness as a staircase, then up at the top of the stairs is 'wide awake', down at the bottom is 'fast asleep' and about halfway down is the state of hypnosis.

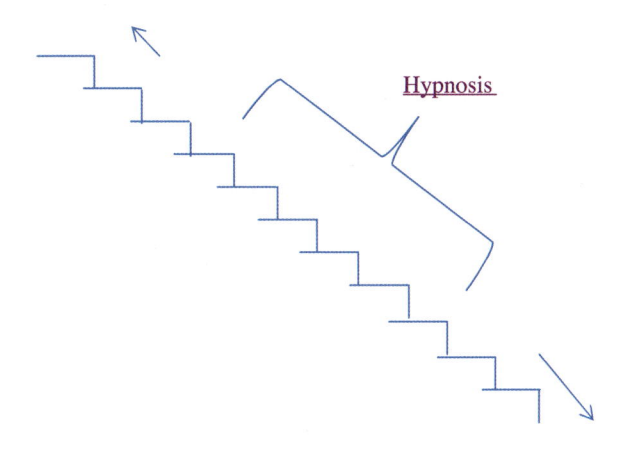

Hypnosis

Did you know that we actually all go through hypnosis at least twice a day, just before waking and just before falling asleep. You may have noticed that some days you get up feeling wide awake and on others you feel sluggish as though you are not as awake and energised, but still conscious. We experience hypnosis naturally in our daily lives:

- Have you ever been lying in bed, hearing your phone bleep with a text message but you just cannot be bothered to take a look at it?
- Have you ever driven from A to B and then wondered how you got there?
- Have you been watching TV and found yourself totally absorbed, perhaps getting upset even though you know it is only a TV programme? It is because you are relaxed, in a form of hypnosis, allowing your imagination to open. You can even get up, go to the loo, come back and slip straight back into this state.
- Adverts – this is why advertising can be so effective. If I ask you to name a breakfast cereal brand, what comes to mind? Did you think Kellogg's? The advertisers catch you while you are in a suggestive state!

Can anyone be hypnotised?
To be hypnotised all you have to do is follow some simple instructions. There are only two types of people who cannot be hypnotised:
- Those with certain serious mental disorders.
- People with very low concentration levels who cannot follow instructions.

So yes, you will be able to hypnotise clients and help them make positive changes that can transform their lives. Isn't that wonderful, and remains my passion and excitement for hypnotherapy.

Clinical Hypnosis simply means delivering scripts, by giving direct and indirect suggestions to help clients with those changes.

My golden rules

These are my golden rules and the first is pretty controversial, I know.

1. Do not complicate things. It does not take hours and hours to learn how to be a hypnotherapist if we keep it simple and follow certain procedures.*

2. I teach a simple formula introducing hypnosis to a client and allowing them to experience the wonderful feeling of relaxing.

3. Then I facilitate change using different techniques to fit the client – not the therapist. Every person is an individual and must be treated as such. You will need to have several different techniques in your toolbox.

4. Finally, almost everyone has lost confidence somewhere along the way, so you must build your client's confidence and give them their own power to choose.

* Though it certainly takes a significant amount of training (and experience) to know how to provide appropriate therapy, as this book will show you.

A word of caution: clients often know what they want and we are there as facilitators to help them achieve it. We need to mediate not arbitrate! It is crucial not to lead a client and assume (wrongly) what they have come to deal with. I always start my first session with a new client by spending ten minutes asking what they want. It is so easy to talk about what we do not want. That is why I include a question on my intake form that says, 'What do you want to achieve with hypnotherapy?' It helps your client to focus on what they hope to achieve. I have included a sample form in the appendix.

Let us begin with the first stage in hypnotherapy. It is called the Induction, where you bring your client into a state of hypnosis.

The Induction

Hypnotherapists use different types of induction but I prefer the slow (progressive) relaxation method. I like it because it takes the average person 12 minutes to relax and this method allows them the time to do so.

Other types of Induction include:
- Rapid Inductions
- Mental Confusion Inductions
- Analytical Inductions
- Metronome Inductions

We will take a look at a couple of these in Chapter Nine, but remember that people like the comfort of familiarity, so it is important that you keep to the same Induction with them and do not keep switching it around. (Just like you do not dye your hair a different colour every time they come to see you. At least, you probably do not!)

On my training course I teach a relaxation induction and use it all through training so people get really confident and comfortable with it. I do not insist they learn if off by heart as that comes naturally with time. I am more interested in teaching how to deliver an Induction with feeling, emphasising words and guiding the client to relaxing and slowing down.

PROGRESSIVE RELAXATION
"Take a nice deep breath and just close your eyes.

Now I want you to notice your breathing ...notice how it feels to slow your breathing down *(Pause)*. Now notice your feet ...toes ...just allow them to relax *(Pause)*. Now allow that relaxation to flow, up your ankles ...calves ...thighs ...just let your legs feel loose limp and relaxed...... *(Pause)*. Notice your stomach and you may find a comfort, growing inside you..........that's right. Now let that comfort flow up your chest *(Pause)*, across your shoulders, down your arms, hands, fingers. Notice your neck, all those little muscles in the back of your neck, just allow your neck to feel comfortable, relaxed. Let that relaxation flow to your head, forehead, eyes, mouth *(Pause)* and as you continue to relax in this way I will count slowly up to seven and as this count progresses you will find that you get tired and sleepy...............

And it doesn't matter if your mind wanders onto more pleasant things. It doesn't even matter if you lose awareness altogether. All that matters now is your own relaxation. So just be comfortable. Settle yourself right down and just let yourself drift gently and easily into that relaxation as I count slowly up to seven. I will start that count for you now.

ONE, relax....
And already you can feel yourself calming down. Becoming much more relaxed now. More and more relaxed. More and more relaxed.

TWO, relax....
You are feeling comfortable. Beginning to feel peaceful too. Just feel that relaxation working its way through your body. Bringing every part of you to rest. Settling yourself right down.

THREE, relax....
And now just breathe a little slower, and deeper now. And each deep breath you take is making you more and more relaxed. More and more relaxed.

FOUR, relax....
Just feel your whole body getting heavier and heavier now. Almost as though you are sinking pleasantly down. Just sinking down into

sheer comfort. As each deep breath you take relaxes you more... and more... and more.

FIVE, relax....
You are feeling drowsier and drowsier ... tired and sleepy ... heavy and relaxed ... beautifully relaxed. Peaceful, sleepy, relaxed.

SIX, relax....
Every part of your body is coming to rest now. Just settling down now. Just settling down into sheer comfort – feeling tired ... sleepy ... relaxed. Tired ... sleepy ... relaxed.

SEVEN, relax....

Just continue drifting now ... deeper and deeper into that relaxation. And I am going to leave you in silence now, just for a few moments, so you can settle yourself right down. And when I talk to you again in a few moments' time, you will be much more relaxed, far more relaxed than you are now. So just rest quietly for the next few moments, until you hear my voice again.

But in the meantime, even the loudest of noises will not concern you, or disturb you in any way. Even the loudest of bangs will not have any importance for you. All that is important now is your own relaxation. So just rest quietly now, until you hear my voice again, in a few moments' time.
(You should be at about ten minutes)

AT LEAST ONE MINUTE OF SILENCE HERE

Okay, as I now slowly count from one to five, just let yourself drift, deeper and deeper, more and more, into that relaxation.

1....2......3........4..........5 *(note increase time between counts)*

Just rest and relax now, that's right, just rest and relax..."

The keys to an effective Induction

- You have to slow your speaking right down.
- Start the first sentence conversationally, and then begin to gradually slow down. Once you slow down you will notice you start to relax. When you are at a nice pace, maintain this. Do not speed up.
- Convey feeling and emotion in your voice avoid monotone.
- You are trying to guide them towards relaxing. Your voice should carry that feeling.
- Diction. You should not make an effort to speak perfect English or change the way you talk. If you have an accent keep it, if you drop your H's continue to do so. Speak naturally. Clients will already be accustomed to your normal way of speaking; to change it would sound false.
- Ensure your voice is not a monotone. Intonation, a rise and fall in your voice, will help to induce trance.
- Lengthen certain words e.g. hazier and hazier, more and more.
- Sit upright so that your diaphragm is open.

Guidelines for using your Induction script

- It should take close to 2 minutes 45 seconds to reach the end of the first three paragraphs and the start of the first count.
- Take a full breath on both sides of each count e.g. (breath) – one – (breath)
- 9 minutes should have passed before you begin the minute's silence.
- During the minute's silence the client slips into their own mind as they relax, so when you start to speak you must come in very quietly, take a full breath in, let out half a breath and then say, 'Okay' before continuing with, 'As I slowly count…'
- On the count to five, increase the length of pauses as the count progresses; it may help to count in your mind

between each number, increasing the count with each increment.
- The Induction should take around 12 minutes from start to finish.

This progressive relaxation induction is a fantastic tool to use.

A word about scripts ...

Good scripts are really useful and I still use them today. Some books and trainers knock scripts and tell you to avoid them. I take a different view. Scripts are not the actual therapy; they are part of the process. Whether you are given full scripts or outlines on your training course, the fact is we all like to know where to go. If you have a good selection of scripts that are tried and tested it allows you time as a therapist to practise and find what works for you. A good training course will give you a good selection of scripts and teach you how to deliver a script in a professional manner.

After all, we use a script for life, whenever you start a new job or learning you have to practise. I remember when I first started using a computer I did not have a clue: the only thing I could do was use the keyboard because I was a typist. I practised and wrote notes to myself to remind me what to do. When I opened my coffee shop the Magick Bean, I learned how to operate the coffee machine by writing notes again. The truth is we all follow a procedure until we learn it off by heart. I like to think of it as our own personal script for life.

As a hypnotherapist, a script means you can get on with facilitating change rather than worry about using clever metaphors. It is what I mean about being client centred – focusing on making a real difference to their life.

Just one word of advice: it is far better to commit your scripts to memory rather than rely on reading them out to your clients.

Personal view: WOW!

Practising inducing hypnosis on my first afternoon training with Lorraine was quite a WOW moment! I'd thought it would take weeks to reach that point. I used to be in a pretty mundane job within a large blue-chip bank. I wanted to learn more about hypnotherapy to find out whether I could 'do the job' as a career change and tie in with my interest in wellbeing and psychology. Lorraine is really inspirational and her knowledge is both full of depth and breadth. It took me a while to acclimatise to Lorraine's relaxed approach to learning, having come from a very corporate background, but now I cannot imagine anything else as it was that individual and tailored approach that enabled me to benefit most.

Alan Sheppard, Hypnotherapist,
NLP Practitioner, Hypno-Gastric Band Specialist

Intonation

The relaxation script should sound like you are telling a story. Imagine you are telling a story to a child you want to fall asleep. Remember to put feeling and intonation into the words to make them come alive.

Noises

Hypnosis is a hard state to break, so even a noise will not bring your client out of this state. In fact you can use the noise (such as heavy rain or a creaky radiator) to help them slip deeper into hypnosis. Following the noise ask them to take a nice deep breath and relax. You can go on to say, 'I just want you to become aware of the noises in the room (refer to them specifically if you like) and just let go as you go deeper and deeper into relaxation / hypnosis.'

Music

Music in a therapy room can be useful if there is likely to be a lot of background noise. They will hear the gentle sound of music rather than different noises. If you wish to play music quietly in the background during hypnosis it is important that you choose something nondescript. Music is a personal thing and just because you like it, it does not mean the client will. Take care with your choice.

Examples of sounds to avoid and why:
- Rain and thunder – fear of thunderstorms
- Sound of birds, nature – they may be scared of the woods
- Pan Pipes – they may dislike the sound

Settling your client before hypnosis

It is important to make sure your client is comfortable before Induction.
- Use a comfortable chair; a recliner is ideal.
- Provide cushions if this helps them feel more comfortable.
- Always cover them with a clean blanket. This not only keeps them warm during hypnosis it also protects their modesty as they relax. A blanket also helps bring a comforting, relaxed feeling.
- Let them know that it is okay if they need to move at all during the process to make themselves more comfortable.
- Have a pack of tissues at hand. Sometimes hypnosis can bring with it emotion and tears. We will cover this in more detail later.
- Ensure your client's arms or legs are not crossed or fingers clasped as this will impede their relaxation. (They might also get pins and needles.)

Recognising the trance state / gauging depth

As you become more experienced you will be able to recognise the tell-tale signs that show a client is in hypnosis. The indicators are:
- With the relaxation of hypnosis, breathing slows down – watch their chest.
- People swallow as they are slipping into hypnosis or going deeper.
- Fluttering of the eyelids / rapid eye movement.

- The face relaxes into an expressionless appearance, which some call the 'hypnotic mask'.
- Often when a client enters hypnosis they will expel air in a long deep breath, often referred to as the 'hypnotic sigh'.
- Some clients flush or go red in the face, neck or chest.

Awakening

At the end of the hypnosis session we need, of course, to awaken the client. You can just simply count from one to seven or you can use an awakening script. I would suggest you do use a script. These have more detail and it is more comfortable and pleasurable to be brought round slowly, particularly if the client has been quite deep in hypnosis. We all know how uncomfortable it can feel if we are suddenly woken from a nap, feeling startled, disorientated and even perhaps a little dizzy.

Ideally the awakening script should last at least 30 – 45 seconds. This awakening script from the pioneer of client-centred hypnotherapy Charles Tebbetts is a particularly good one.

AWAKENING SCRIPT

"Now I am going to count from one up to five and slowly awaken you (add here a suggestion connected with their therapy, such as feeling positive and determined to be a non-smoker).

ONE, slowly, calmly, easily and gently you are returning to your full awareness once again.

TWO, every muscle and nerve in your body feels loose, limp and relaxed and you feel wonderfully good.

THREE, you feel perfect in every way. Physically perfect, mentally alert and emotionally serene, and when you awaken from this trance state you are perfect in every way, responding appropriately to each and all situations.

FOUR, eyes sparkling just as though they have been bathed in spring water. On the next number now let your eyelids open.

FIVE, eyelids open, you are fully aware once again. Take a good deep breath and s-t-r-e-t-c-h."

Voice Modulation
While you are delivering an awakening script, raise your pitch or volume and slightly increase your tempo. If awakening is done in a monotone voice then a client that is in a deep state may not respond.

What happens if they do not open their eyes and wake up?
- Do not worry! All that will happen is that they will drift off into a pleasant sleep.
- Tell them, 'I know you are enjoying a really pleasurable experience however if you do not wake up now you will never be able to enjoy this peace, comfort and security in my office ever again, so it is imperative you wake up on my count of 7.' Then dramatically increase your voice volume, speed and pitch as you count.

On awakening – time to 'come round'
The hypnotic state is not an easy state to break, so it is important you make sure there is plenty of time for your client to come around fully before leaving your office. Allow at least 10 minutes. This time post hypnosis is your chance to:
- Check the client has understood everything you have done and talk through what took place.
- Explain that you will give them a recording of the session and that they should listen to it every day.
- Make the next appointment.

Why should we check the client has understood everything that has taken place?
- You can never be sure how deep they have gone. They may be a somnambulist, someone who drops so deeply into hypnosis that they are out cold and have no recollection of anything that has happened.
- It is important for their therapy that they are aware of what has taken place and have an idea of what will happen next.
- It is important that the customer feels secure, knowing what has happened helps this.

You will give all clients a recording to listen to, if possible, every day from now until their next session. It is important they do this as it will reinforce their initial therapy and add to the benefits of the next session.

Practising hypnotherapy

As well as reading this book, practising hypnotherapy is an important aspect of your learning. It allows you to:
- Put yourself in your client's shoes.
- Understand some of your client's experiences.
- Discover what works well and what does not.
- Grow your understanding and appreciation of hypnosis.
- Experience for yourself the benefits of hypnosis, building your belief and confidence in the therapy.
- Allay any apprehensions you may have as a hypnotherapist, e.g. experiencing interruptions or noise.

Do make sure your trainer is still actively practising as a hypnotherapist so they are not out of touch with the way people talk, feel and react.

Advice on recording software and equipment

During your training you may need to make a recording of an induction and a relaxation:
- As part of your assessment.
- As part of your case study practical work.
- To issue to your clients.

You can use free software packages that are available for download from the internet or invest at some point in other packages that allow further functionality, quality and flexibility.

You will need to invest in a microphone headset. These are available online at quite reasonable prices.

Recommended microphone
Plantronics Blackwire C610.

Free recording software
Audacity.

Other Recording Software
NCH Wave Pad – This comes as a bundle that includes a recording pad, express burn and wavepad software for adding music as a background.

Recording tips
- To ensure good sound quality, place the microphone below your mouth to avoid the p…p…p sound.
- If, when you listen back to your recording you discover a whooshing sound, check that the speakers/volume are not too loud.
- To check the quality of the recording you need to play it back on a separate sound system as a recording can sound very different to when you play it back on a computer.

NOTE – Insurance
You will be involved in lots of practical work with clients during your training and as you progress and begin to feel confident you may decide you would like to start charging your clients. If you are taking money for your service you must have insurance. You can find out more about this from the General Hypnotherapy Register.

Test yourself

How could you describe hypnosis? *half way between being wide awake & fast asleep*

Who cannot be hypnotised? *those with certain mental disorders. People with low concentration who cannot follow instructions*

How long does it take the average person to relax? *12 mins*

Name two types of Induction. *slow progressive relaxation method, rapid induction*

List four things that are important in the delivery of the Induction. *1. slow speaking down 2. lengthen certain words - hazier & hazier, relax & more & more 3. avoid monotone 4. if you are trying to guide them towards relaxing, your voice should carry that feeling*

How do you recognise the trance state? List three indicators. *Breathing slows down, rapid eye movement, face relaxes*

Give two reasons why you should spend time chatting with your client following hypnosis. *① you are never sure how deeply they have gone. They may drop so deeply into relaxation that they are outcold & have no recollection of anything that has happened ② It is important that the client feels secure, knowing what has happened helps*

Give two reasons why is it important to provide your clients with recordings?

Analytical People

Some hypnotherapists are frightened of working with analytical people. I hear lots of talk about how hard it is for them to go into hypnosis and what difficult clients they are. Rubbish! That is an insult to people's intelligence.

Personally I love working with so-called analytical people. In my experience all they need to do is understand what it is that they want and how to get it. They will do the rest. As I have explained, it is not difficult to go into hypnosis: we drop in and out of hypnosis all day, every day. Having learned my simple, straightforward progressive Induction really well, you can be confident that it is 100% successful. More to the point, I feel that if you are confident about what you do and really understand what hypnosis is, then every client will have an enjoyable experience and will just drift gently into hypnosis.

When a client says to me that they weren't hypnotised (which is very rare these days), I will be thinking to myself, 'Well how do you know?' Out loud, of course, I talk about how well they took my suggestions and what we call arm assurance, a way of gauging whether someone is in hypnosis that we will come into in Chapter Three. I am a great believer in keeping things simple: in hypnosis, all your client has to be able to do is follow simple instructions.

Let me tell you about Maude. She was a lovely colourful lady in her 80s who came to me because she had a fear of thunder. This fear was so bad that she was reading the shipping reports. Now, we are in England so we have very few big thunderstorms.

When I was chatting to her she started telling me all about her family, how she was the baby of three sisters and how she never really took much interest in the middle sister Margaret. Yet when Margaret died Maude discovered amazing paintings and a book her sister had written, and realised she had never had the pleasure of really knowing her sister.

Eventually I started the induction I knew so well. Talking slowly, I got to the part where I said, 'You are feeling very, very relaxed.' Maude opened her eyes and looked at me and said, 'No I am not!' And she wasn't, which really made me smile. So I asked her to close her eyes and I tried a children's Induction as the progressive relaxation was so obviously not for Maude.

I said: Maude, I want you to imagine that you are sitting down outside, somewhere comfortable and relaxed. Have you done that?

Maude: If you say so, Lorraine.
Me: Okay, now I want you to imagine you have some balloons in your hand. Have you done that?
Maude: Yes.
Me: What colour or colours are the balloons?
Maude: Oh, now you want me to give them a colour!!!

By now the appointment had gone on for nearly two hours and for the first time I thought to myself, 'I cannot do this, I think I will tell her.' Then I noticed on my desk a paper from a hypnosis conference. It said in bold letters, 'Chasing rainbows – if all else fails, make it up.' So I abandoned my plan and said: 'Maude, I want you to imagine you are standing outside your home. Can you do that?'

Maude: Yes.
Me: What colour is your front door?
Maude: Red.
Me: Okay, I want you to go inside. Go into your lounge and sit down comfortably. Have you done that?
Maude: Yes.
Me: Now I want you to imagine that Margaret is there. Can you see her?
Maude: Yes.
Me: Now I want you to talk to Margaret. Tell her all that you need to say and when you have done that, just let me know.

Maude went straight into rapid eye movement (REM), a state of deep hypnosis. I felt so honoured to witness this – it was brilliant. Maude dealt with the issues she had for not getting to know her sister better, then we moved on to her main reason for coming to see me. I talked to her subconscious mind, saying that Maude had come to me to deal with her fear of thunder and could it make the necessary adjustments? I waited and when it was all confirmed using the IMR finger technique we will cover in Chapter Four, I counted Maude up out of hypnosis and off she went.

When I worked with Maude I worked from the Magick Bean my coffee shop, where I had a little room in the back I called Room 101. A couple of months later, this lovely lady came into my shop and announced in her wonderful flamboyant manner: 'Lorraine darling, I have told my doctor about you and told him he should have some hypnosis. It is wonderful.' Her fear of thunderstorms was gone.

How great is that?

Chapter Two

The Holistic Theory of Man

The Conscious and the Subconscious

To really understand hypnosis and how it works we need to consider what 'man' is, how he (or she) is made up, the parts that combine together to create the whole, fully functioning human being.

The Two-Part Theory of Man – the medical profession's viewpoint

The medical profession traditionally see 'man' as having two distinct parts:
1. The Physical Body – defined as the skeleton, the muscles, the organs, the pipe-work and the skin that covers the whole.

2. The Brain and Nervous System.

Medical professionals see the mind as part and parcel of the brain and nervous system. They see it as a physical element and as such use physical means to treat psychological problems. Examples are

ECT, lobotomies and psychoactive drug therapy, such as pills for depression or anxiety.

The hypnotherapist's view is that there is far more to it than that.

The Holistic Theory of Man – the hypnotherapist's viewpoint

1. The Physical Body – defined as the skeleton, the muscles, the organs, the pipe-work and the skin that covers the whole.

2. The Brain and Nervous System.

3. The Energy Body – our chakras and auras.

4. The Mind – comprised of the conscious and subconscious.

What is the Energy Body?
Many alternative practitioners work with the energy body. Examples are:
- Reiki therapists
- Massage therapists
- Acupuncture
- Aura reading and mapping
- Tai Chi

The aura is an energy field surrounding our body. As it can now be photographed, its existence is accepted by science. When you have alternative treatments your chakras are balanced and your aura is healed, bringing with it a feeling of wellbeing.

What is the Mind?
It is the mind that operates the brain: the mind is the 'controller'. The brain/nervous system and the energy body are communicators

between the mind and the body, carrying out the mind's instructions, providing the pathways to put in motion everything that happens in all parts of the body. If you would like an analogy, the brain can be likened to a computer. It is the tool that carries out functions only once it has been set in motion by the user (the mind.)

The conscious and the subconscious mind

The human being is an organism living in an environment. We receive stimuli from that environment and we produce responses to them. Humans respond either physically, mentally or both physically and mentally.

The mediator between the stimulus and the response is the mind, which means our mental and physical reactions are the result of the mind's behaviour.

The mind is made up of two separate parts, the conscious mind and the subconscious mind.

The Conscious Mind – operates anything that requires 'conscious' effort. We are aware of the instructions it is issuing. It fires actions and operates analytical functions such as thinking, questioning and reasoning.

The Subconscious Mind – conversely the subconscious mind controls functions that are not the result of conscious thought. It has three main functions:
1. Operation and maintenance of the physical body.

2. Storage of our skills and habits.

3. Storage of all our memories.

1. Operation and maintenance of the physical body

To help us understand this let us consider what happens when we go to sleep at night. The moment we drift into sleep we lose all consciousness. It is as though our conscious mind has ceased to exist. When we are asleep it is the subconscious mind that keeps us breathing and our heart beating; it tells us to turn over or wake up to take a drink or go the toilet. So the subconscious mind is in control of our bodily functions; this also happens at microscopic levels, renewing and replacing our cells, liver cells, bone cells, skin cells, etc.

2. Storage of our skills and habits

Many of the things we do require no conscious effort at all – we do them automatically. Consider walking for example: do you know which foot you start with or how many paces you take? No, of course not, because all you do consciously is initiate the action and everything else that happens is automatic. The same is true of talking: when you talk you do not think about vocabulary or grammar, you just talk. First learning these skills took a lot of conscious effort but now we have learned these skills so well we no longer have to think about them. The process has transferred from the conscious mind to the subconscious. This is where learnt skills are stored.

3. Storage of all our memories

Memories that are new or important are readily accessible to the conscious mind. All other memories, no matter how old, are stored in the subconscious memory bank. The conscious only has limited access to this store.

So, the subconscious is working 24/7 and does far more than the conscious mind: it operates our heartbeat, repairs our skin if we have cut it, monitors the environment and makes sure we are safe. I also believe we have *unconscious* behaviours, which means we did not learn them consciously. Actually, because the mind so far cannot be seen, pictured or felt, I personally believe it is not in our bodies at all. I think it is too big and just like our auras, which can now be photographed, I think the mind is outside our bodies. I believe the way we think can actually change what is happening in our world and if we think positively then positive things will happen.

This is fundamental, so I will say it again: positive thinking makes positive things happen.
That is the joy of hypnotherapy, and why I get so much pleasure out of my work.

We are now going to go into some more detail about how the mind works in response to stimuli from the environment, and it may be useful to look at the following diagrams.

How the mind works

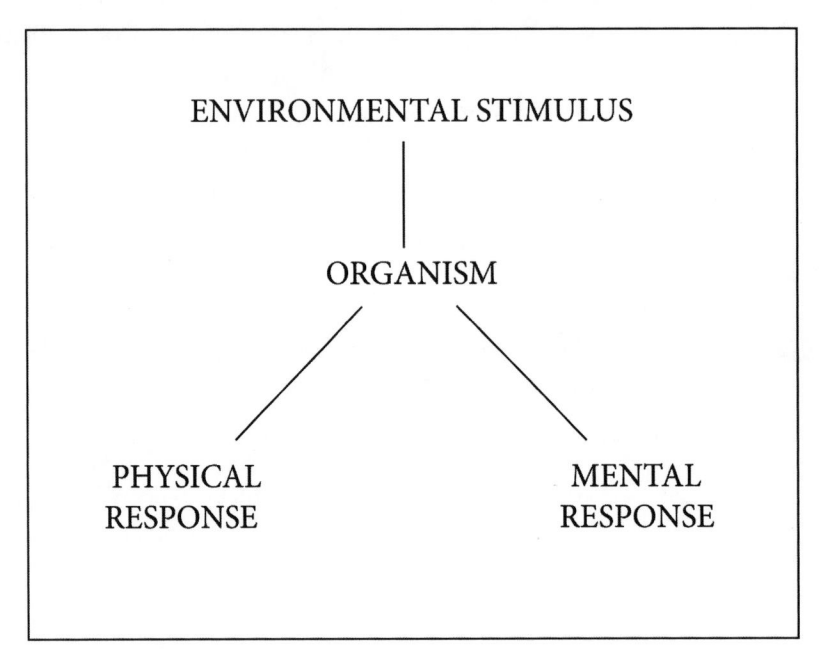

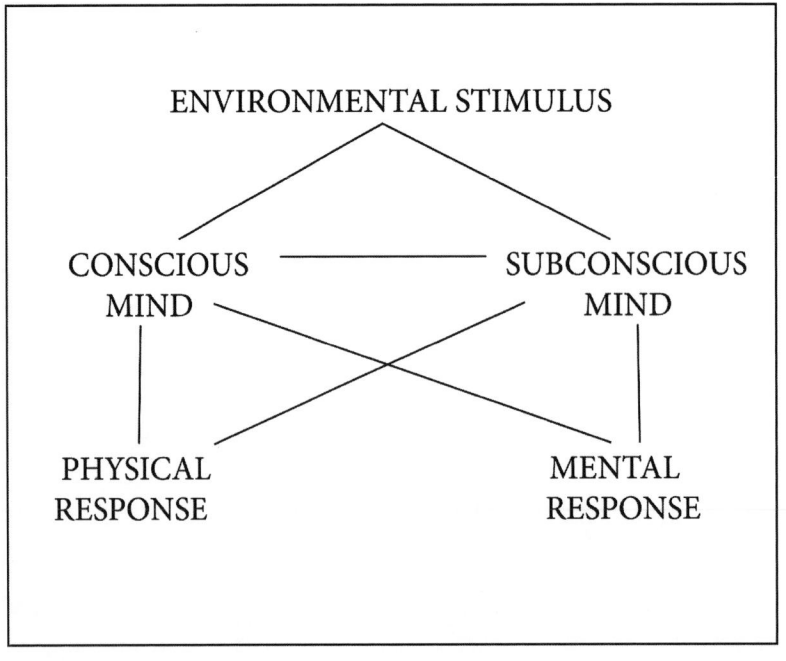

```
            ENVIRONMENTAL STIMULUS
                      |
                   ORGANISM
                   /       \
           PHYSICAL        MENTAL
           RESPONSE        RESPONSE
```

```
            ENVIRONMENTAL STIMULUS
              /                \
       CONSCIOUS  ———————  SUBCONSCIOUS
         MIND                   MIND
           |    \    /           |
           |     \  /            |
           |      \/             |
           |      /\             |
       PHYSICAL              MENTAL
       RESPONSE              RESPONSE
```

Which perceives stimuli – the conscious or subconscious?

Conscious mind example – Frequently we use our ability to focus all our attention on just one sense: when listening to music, for instance. We may close our eyes to focus on listening to the music; this is a conscious action.

Subconscious mind example – Imagine you are in bed asleep. Through the night the temperature changes, becoming cooler. What happens? You wake up because you feel cold. The coldness must have been perceived subconsciously, because you were not aware of it until you woke up.

So both the conscious and subconscious perceive stimuli.

Which responds to stimuli – the conscious or the subconscious?

We saw in the top diagram how we can respond physically or mentally or both physically and mentally to stimuli. Now let us go further.

Conscious mind example – If you are asked a question, you think about it, reason it out and give a reply. The thinking and reasoning is done with full awareness therefore it is a *conscious, mental response*. The response requires the manipulation of the mouth and vocal cords and this is a *conscious physical response*. So the conscious mind can respond both physically and mentally.

Subconscious mind example – One of the stimuli that we can receive from the environment is stress. Stress takes many forms but in this instance let us imagine that you suddenly find yourself in a very dangerous position. Under these circumstances a very special part of the nervous system comes into action without any conscious control. It causes you to produce adrenaline, making your pupils dilate, your mouth go dry, your heart beat to speed up and the blood supply to your muscles to increase. This reaction prepares your body for action so you are more able to cope with the situation. So the subconscious mind must be able to produce a *physical response*.

Stress can also affect our mental state. Conditions such as depression, anxiety and apathy are all reactions to stress. These conditions are not produced consciously in most cases. (Although it would be possible, it is very unlikely you would consciously attempt to produce depression, for instance.) The subconscious mind must therefore be producing a *mental response*.

So both the conscious and subconscious minds respond to stimuli.

Conscious and subconscious – Are they connected? Do they communicate?

To answer this we need to consider memory. Some things we can remember clearly and well, others we cannot remember at all. Sometimes we can work at remembering something and after a period of time it suddenly comes to us. How can we explain this? Let us assume that as events happen to us, they are recorded in some sort of memory bank. They are stored until required for further use. Remembering is simply withdrawing an item from that memory bank.

So, where is that memory bank located? If it were in the conscious mind, we would not have to work to find certain memories and even if we did we would always manage it. It must therefore be located in the subconscious mind.

However, because of the way we use our memories, we have to conclude that the conscious mind must have access to the memory bank. There is therefore a connecting link from the conscious to the subconscious mind. Similarly, we know that there must also be a link from the subconscious to the conscious. There are times when for no apparent reason a memory will suddenly pop into our head. The subconscious mind has fed that memory to the conscious mind. This could not happen unless a link existed.

This is shown in the complete model of how the mind works in the diagram on page 24.

Hypnotherapists work with the subconscious mind, and we have a fascinating profession.

Personal view: The right mindset

I have successfully built and sold two companies and now spend time mentoring other business owners to achieve peak performance. I have always believed that success and failure lie within the mind so I wanted to learn more about the mind. Enrolling with Lorraine is without doubt one of the best things that I have done. I really find using NLP techniques whilst in hypnosis very powerful and Lorraine's teaching has ultimately led to me being a lot more relaxed within myself and believing that with the right mindset anything is possible.

Dave Symondson

The origin of client problems

To recap, when we first learn new skills we need to store and protect them so they are not forgotten. When a child learns to walk, it crawls and stumbles at first, then masters how to stay upright and walk steadily. Once we have mastered this we do not need to think about it consciously, it becomes automatic. We never forget how to walk or unlearn this skill. The same goes for driving, riding a bike and talking. When you pick up an egg or a hammer you do not have to consciously think about what pressure to apply, you just do it. This is because we lock away the skill in our subconscious mind to keep it safe. In fact, we can use the analogy that the subconscious is like a safe, its contents remaining under lock and key.

Unfortunately, as we go through life not all the skills we learn are positive ones. Through repetition, we learn how to be depressed or have panic attacks; we learn a fear of flying, lifts, crowds and so on – in fact creating and locking away these negative skills behind the safe door.

Hypnosis allows us to communicate with the subconscious mind. When we are relaxed, the safe door swings open and the client has access to its contents. We can then help them make positive changes to any learned behaviours they want to get rid of.

Life influences and the creation of unique individuals

Every individual is different because as we go through life our experiences and the influences around us mould our personality and how we react to stimuli. Our experiences are stored and eventually affect how we think and behave. We are influenced by our parents, school, religion, friends, codes of conduct and the things people say and do. These influences create a unique individual, 'warts and all', as we are the product of both positive and negative influences.

The subconscious is not secretive – its main job is to protect us and relieve stress. Unlike the conscious mind it learns without analysing, so if you grow up in an environment where the only way to be heard is to shout and get angry then the subconscious stores this and when you need to be heard you will find that you want to shout or get angry. As far as the subconscious is concerned the problem is dealt with. But if this behaviour is not acceptable to a client, they seek therapy.

The avenues open to the subconscious are both physical and physiological. If you produce a rash when you are stressed, that is what the subconscious learns to do and as far as the subconscious is concerned the problem is dealt with. If you have a migraine when you get worried, again as far as the subconscious is concerned the problem is dealt with. Some of us learn to comfort eat and we can then develop a weight problem. Many of our behaviours we do learn unconsciously, such as the type of people we are attracted to. Some of us are attracted to people who cause us problems: we do not know why we do this, we just do.

The importance of establishing causes

Some hypnotherapists simply take the client into hypnosis and then use a standard script to treat the problem. The pitfalls of this approach are only short-term improvement or no improvement at all.

Why should we establish the cause of the problem?
- All causes are individual, 'one size does not fit all'.
- To deal with it.
- To change response to stimuli and establish new positive response/behaviour.

Unique experiences create unique causes for any client seeking therapy. So to effectively treat a client we need to deal with the cause of the problem. To ignore it would be like using a sticking plaster, a short-lived, temporary measure.

Every client must be dealt with as an individual, as no two people are the product of the same formative influences. Yes, it is a challenge but it also makes our working life stimulating as a hypnotherapist, varied and often fun too.

Test yourself

What is the Holistic Theory of Man? (Four points)

What are the three major functions of the subconscious mind?

Is it always necessary to deal with the cause of the problem?

Behaviours

As we have seen, the subconscious learns from stimuli and what you hear and see can have a big impact. Your parents might have said, 'You must be seen and not heard' or, 'Eat up everything on your plate.' Teachers may say, 'You are not an artist' or, 'You are not very bright.' If you got stuck in a lift as a child you could develop a fear. Yet from every behaviour we have we do somehow get a secondary benefit, no matter how small. For example, if you are unfortunate enough to produce migraines, you do at least get some time to yourself. If you over-eat, you get the satisfaction of the taste of food and you may unconsciously not want to attract a partner into your life; you may also have been insecure as a child and been told that when you get 'big' life will be better. Your subconscious mind might have interpreted this literally.

For some reason, and I do not know why, I had an allergy to metal and could only wear silver. There was no reason for me not to be able to wear costume jewellery but somehow my mind got a mixed message. I had hypnosis and can now wear whatever I want. (I must admit that when I first found I could wear anything, I did go rather mad and looked a bit like a Christmas tree. I consciously changed that and now only wear a small amount of jewellery.)

When we go into hypnosis with a therapist we can find out how we have learned to produce a particular behaviour. Once we have this understanding we can do something about it. The subconscious is not a truth drug – it is our perception of the world and we all model our world differently. It is like a bright nine-year-old, learning and changing all the time.

If we have suffered for a long time with our problem, it is part of us, and it is so important to learn how to live without it – this is something you will have to help your clients with carefully. Once their problem is resolved, they must suffer with the void it leaves behind.

Chapter Three

Suggestibility

The Finger Test

Suggestion

The Language of Hypnosis

Arm Assurance

In this chapter we are going to look at the finger test, a technique we use with clients before hypnosis, then move on to the language of the subconscious, the ways that we communicate during hypnosis. The finger test is a simple way to help your client relax and to help build a rapport with them.

Purpose of the finger test
- The finger test is used to demonstrate to your client how easy it is to follow an instruction.
- Clients are often a little nervous at their first session and completing this exercise helps to give them confidence and belief as they see how easy it is to listen and follow your instructions.

- It is also a tool for you as the therapist because you can find out prior to hypnosis if your client easily responds to your instructions or blocks them at some level. If they struggle with the finger test they may need a little extra work to go into hypnosis, so with this knowledge you can be prepared. We will discuss what you need – a deepener – in Chapter Four.

THE FINGER TEST

Ask your client to hold their hands in front of them, at eye level, with their fingers interlocked and elbows bent. Now tell them to extend their index fingers towards the ceiling and to separate the ends so that they are about an inch apart. Tell them to squeeze all the fingers together except for their index fingers. Show them what to do.

Say:

"Now fix your gaze on the gap between your index fingers and relax those fingers as you do so.

Now just notice that gap getting smaller.

You will find your fingers moving together.

In a few moments your fingers will touch.

As soon as they touch you will feel them pressing against each other, you may even start to see a little whiteness in the skin where the fingers are joined.

Now fingers together, the pressure is building, see that whiteness.

As you continue to stare at those fingers I want to show you something.

Think about what is happening, the fingers come together quite naturally and now they are pressing against each other.

If you wanted to separate them, you would have to do it consciously, wouldn't you?

Now I will show you something. I am just going to count up to 3 and when I reach the count of 3 you will find, that without you doing anything, those fingers will just drift apart as naturally as they came together.

As I count now, just watch it happen.

One you can feel the pressure coming off now two you can see the colour returning three.

Yes, that's right, now as you look at those fingers you can feel the pressure easing, releasing. You can see the colour coming back as that pressure releases.

Rather than being a pressure, it now becomes a gentle touch and in a moment you will find they are actually separated and you can see daylight between those fingers as they continue to drift back to their original position."

In all cases the fingers will have at least come together at the beginning; however some clients may not part their fingers to complete the exercise. The finger test might not work successfully in this way if the client is blocking you and not going with your instructions.

What to do if the fingers do not part
If the fingers do not part, say:
'That's right, now in a moment I am going to touch your hands and gently lower them into your lap. And you will find yourself relaxing, feeling peaceful and relaxed. And I wonder if you choose to just let your eyes close or keep them open. I wonder what you will feel most comfortable with.'

Why the finger test works
1. As a person gazes at the gap between their fingers it becomes difficult to maintain focus and their eyes will automatically become blurry or hazy.

2. When you hold your fingers in this way, with your other fingers clasped together, it is natural for your fingers to want to move together.

3. It is not natural for your fingers to separate so your subconscious will perform what you ask, going into learning mode, just in case you have to do this for the rest of your life.

4. The client is given a direct suggestion during the process, 'You will find your fingers will just drift apart.'

Practising your first client visit
During your training, you should have plenty of opportunities to practise client visits.

Role-play should be an important part of this training, and I am providing here an example of an exercise you can carry out with a partner. One of you plays the client, the other the therapist.

At the start of the visit the therapist will need to:
- Establish / clarify the client's problem.
- Establish what they know about hypnosis.
- Briefly explain what hypnosis is.
- Carry out the finger test.

ASK: What is it you would like to achieve from hypnosis?

PARAPHRASE the client's response to confirm understanding: 'So what you would like to achieve from hypnosis is...'

REASSURE your client that you can help: 'When you are relaxed in hypnosis that is when your imagination opens and as the therapist I can then help you to make the positive changes you want.'

ROLE-PLAY ONE

Client's brief:

Initial Statement of Problem – You have come here today for help with the following problem:

- You suffer with anxiety as a passenger in a car.
- You are aged 19 (provide this information only if asked the question.)

Information the therapist needs to establish through delving deeper with a further question:

- When you were learning to drive with your dad you pulled out at a junction and had an accident.
- Your immediate priority now is to be able to get into a car without panicking (you are not focusing on learning to drive yet).

What you know about hypnosis:

- You have seen Paul McKenna on TV.
- You have seen a stage hypnotist, where a friend of yours went on stage and did funny things.

ROLE-PLAY TWO

Client's brief:

Initial Statement of Problem – You have come here today for help with the following problem:
- You have a problem sleeping.
- You are aged 55 (provide this information only if asked the question.)

Information the therapist needs to establish through delving deeper with a further question:
- You struggle with actually falling asleep at night.
- You also wake up during the night and then cannot get back to sleep.
- The problem is affecting your quality of life as during the day you go to work feeling tired and irritable.
- Your aim is to be able to fall asleep easily when going to bed and sleep comfortably through the night.

What you know about hypnosis:
- A friend came to see the therapist to give up smoking and hypnosis worked for them.

Discuss with your partner afterwards what worked, what you found difficult and what you could change in the future.

Suggestion – the language of hypnosis

It is time to think about the words we use to communicate with the subconscious. First we are going to understand the two key types of suggestion, Direct Suggestion and Indirect Suggestion. Both types of suggestion are powerful in their own right and each has their strengths with specific types of therapy and different personality types.

Direct suggestion

Direct suggestions are also sometimes known as authoritarian or paternal suggestions. Direct suggestion involves actually giving a client a command, telling them what to do or be.

Examples:
- You are a non-smoker.
- You feel calm and relaxed.
- You will listen to my voice and as you listen to my voice you will relax as I count from 10 to 1.
- You will now see yourself as a self-confident person.
- Your eyes become heavier and heavier.

Clinical Hypnosis uses direct and indirect suggestion involving the delivery of standard scripts.

Indirect suggestion

Indirect suggestions are also sometimes known as permissive or maternal suggestions. Indirect suggestion uses a lot of imagery and metaphor requiring the client to use their imagination.
Examples:
If you had a client with a brain tumour an example of indirect suggestion would be getting him to focus inside on what is happening in his body, asking what would it look like? How would it feel? Allowing him to visualise the healing antibodies in his own way.

The 20th century American psychiatrist and hypnotherapist Milton Erickson favoured and perfected this technique, taking a poetic or creative approach, creating a story to represent the client's challenge and goal. With one client who was a keen gardener and wary of hypnosis, he told a story about the life of a growing tomato plant, using it as a metaphor for dealing with pain and recovery from illness.

The use of stories for hypnosis goes back a long way. In 1774 a woman's son developed a tumour that had to be removed surgically. The mother sat beside him during surgery and told him a story so interesting that the young boy felt no pain in spite of the fact that no anaesthesia was available then. The surgery was successful. Many years later the boy published the story his mother had told him. His name was Jacob Grimm and the story was 'Snow White.'

Remember the story of the ugly duckling, that no one loved who turned into a beautiful swan? He did not know it and thought he was ugly until he saw himself in the mirror. You can use stories like that of the ugly duckling as a metaphor for your client's transformation into a beautiful and confident person, shedding all the ugliness and low self-esteem of the past.

Indirect suggestion can also be more subtle (without use of imagery). Rather than using a direct suggestion the client is given the illusion of choice by deciding whether they will carry out the action requested by the therapist.

Compare the following two suggestions:

Direct Suggestion: 'Your eyes become heavier and heavier.'
Indirect Suggestion: '...and you might discover that your eyes are becoming heavier and heavier.'

This type of suggestion is less obvious, less likely to be met with resistance and so it could be useful with clients who are more analytical or do not respond well to the authoritative approach of direct suggestion.

Most hypnosis makes use of both direct and indirect suggestion. Some people respond more to the direct approach while others respond more effectively when it is less apparent. In general, you will find the majority of clients respond well to both.

The Four Rules Governing Suggestion

Now we understand the types of suggestion let us take a look at the four rules to follow with the use of all suggestions.

1. All suggestions should be POSITIVE (focusing on the positive goal, rather than what your client should 'not' do or be.)

Example:
- POSITIVE – 'You will sleep easily.'
- NEGATIVE – 'You will not toss and turn in your sleep.'

This does not mean that the word 'not' cannot ever be used, but rather that it is more effective to focus on 'what you want' rather than 'what you do not want'.

2. Use plenty of REPETITION.
For us to learn anything we have to repeat it over and over again, and this concept also applies to learning in hypnosis.

If you tell someone they are stupid / attractive enough times they will believe it.

If you tell someone they will sleep easily enough times they will believe it.

3. Whenever possible use VISUALISATION.
This means to imagine a picture, to visualise the current situation and alter it until it meets your requirements. For instance, if your client has a physical problem, then ask them to imagine they can see inside their body and see what is wrong. Then put it right. Imagine the way it FEELS rather than the way it IS. In other words, they do not need anatomical knowledge for this. If it is helpful for them to see the inside of their body in a way that the client can relate to for example a computer programmer may be able to visualise running an anti-virus and removing the problem.

If they cannot find a picture of the actual situation, then find an analogy from which you can extract principles. To improve study for instance, they could imagine their brain as being like a bathroom sponge, soaking up knowledge in the same way a sponge soaks up water. Pictures add power: if the mind can see it, it is true. Have you heard of the law of the mind? It says that, 'What the mind can believe, it can achieve.' Einstein said, 'Knowledge is what we know now, imagination encompasses all there is to know.'

4. Be PATIENT
Do not always expect instant results. Behaviours and habits perfected over years can take some time before change sets in. Remember the saying: 'The impossible, we do at once. Miracles take a little longer!'

The Language of Hypnosis
Now let us take a look at some of the language we use in hypnosis and why. There are certain words that the subconscious loves and using these effectively will bring the results we are hoping for.

FIND
Use of the word **'find'** in hypnosis produces a direct suggestion. It is a really positive word because the child inside us loves to find things. Remember when you were a child, your mother might say to you, "Go on Jan, find your shoes" and so you'd run off, find and produce them and be showered with praise. So it is a word that automatically has good feelings attached to it, praise and reward.
e.g. 'You will now find that your eyes are getting heavier and heavier.'

MORE
You will know from your Induction that the word 'more' is used a lot.
e.g. 'You become more and more relaxed.'
Use of the word **'more'** is effective because the mind naturally likes to grow things. Again it is a really positive word

NOTICE
When we use the word **'notice'** it is a direct suggestion, when you tell someone to notice something they will automatically pay attention to it.
e.g. 'Notice your breathing.'

NOW
The word **'now'** is used often in hypnosis, it is effective because it is a direct instruction; it gets your attention.
e.g. 'Now, take a nice deep breath.'

TRY

The word **'try'** implies failure to the subconscious, so when you precede a suggestion with 'try' the implication is that it will be difficult or impossible.

e.g. "...imagine your eyelids are glued shut, they are locked so tight that even if you TRY to open them you find that they just lock together tighter and tighter."

THAT'S RIGHT

This is a very powerful phrase. People love to do things right. It is a form of praise and people love to be praised **'that's right'**, it makes them feel good. When a behaviour is praised it encourages more of the same.

e.g. 'That's right, you are doing that beautifully.'

REPETITION OF WORDS

e.g. 'more and more, heavier and heavier, hazier and hazier.

Repetition of words in this way is effective because it makes you focus on the word and action, simply because it is said twice. Saying the word twice reinforces its importance.

TERMINOLOGY TO AVOID

Take care to avoid language or terminology with double meanings or negative connotations. A phrase that is quite natural to you could mean something very different to someone else. For instance, with a phrase like *'sinking down into the comfort of your resting place'* the words 'resting place' could be misinterpreted as meaning the grave. This could obviously create difficulties. 'Sinking down' might be linked to a fear of drowning, so say instead, 'sinking pleasantly down'. It makes sense when you are creating, changing or using a script to continually ask the question 'Could this be interpreted in any other way?'

Remember this language, you are going to be using it a lot, in fact you are going to see it in action in our next technique, the arm assurance procedure.

The Arm Assurance Procedure

The arm assurance procedure is a technique we use with the client on their first session, once they are in hypnosis. It is a technique you have to learn by heart, as you will need to watch your client throughout and adapt to their responses. Here is an outline, but memorise it and remember to use seeing, hearing and feeling words.

ARM ASSURANCE (Outline)

" In a moment I am going to come over by your side and gently lift your (*indicate left or right*) arm in the air. This will not disturb you in any way. I want you now to hold your arm in the air. (*Make this instruction very clear. Some clients are very relaxed and their arm can be very heavy.*)

Repeat.

I want you now to use your imagination. I want you to imagine your arm feels light, so very light, as if it is resting on a cushion of air. I want you to imagine that you can feel me placing some cushions under your arm. That's right, I want you to imagine if they are hard or soft cushions, imagine what colour or colours they are...

Keep going until you feel that their arm is relaxed in the air. Then say:

If you wanted to, you would be able to leave your (*left or right*) arm floating comfortably all day. If you wanted to...

Proceed.

I am now going to lift your (*right or left*) arm in the air again. This will not disturb your relaxation in any way. As I gently lift your (*indicate right or left*) arm in the air, I want you now to notice all you can about your (*right or left*) arm. Feel your fingers, wrist, elbow, upper arm. I want you to notice all you can about this arm.

Now I want you to imagine that I have just placed (*suggest a bucket or bag, whichever you feel most comfortable with*) a bucket in your hand. That's right, just imagine you feel me placing a bucket in your hand … Now, do you remember the sound of sand being poured? That's right, I want you to imagine that you can hear sand and see sand being poured into that bucket. You can feel sand being poured into that bucket and you find that your arm is getting heavier and heavier as it wants to come down and rest. Heavier and heavier.

Keep going until the arm starts to come down.

Try to hold your arm up and you will find the harder you try, the heavier your arm feels...

Keep going until the arm is down.

When the arm is down, take the other arm down.

I want you now to let both your arms feel normal, comfortable and fine.

Repeat. (You must always restore normality.)

I want you to think about what you have just achieved. You know that there was no sand and no bucket … but you took my suggestion and allowed your arm to come down. I want you now to feel assured that when I give you any suggestion, you will be able to take it and do something real with it and make any positive change you want … "

Please be aware that everyone will be different and some people will respond very quickly. Others will take time.

Note the use of particular words. The key words are **hear** the sand, **feel** the sand, **see** the sand. When the arm starts to come down, say, '**Try** to hold your arm up (*the word try implies failure*) and you will **find** (*the subconscious mind loves to find*) your arm gets heavier and heavier as it wants to come down and rest.'

There are a number of benefits from this procedure:
- It is a **'convincer'** – Even though you have explained what hypnosis is and also completed a finger test there is still a part of the client that wants to know that:
  a) They are in hypnosis.
  b) They are doing it right.
  This procedure demonstrates to them how they can follow suggestions and use their imagination to effect change; it convinces them they are in hypnosis.
- The procedure shows you as a therapist **how deep they are in hypnosis.**
- It also helps the person in hypnosis to **go deeper** into the state after experiencing acceptance of the suggestions.

Prior to hypnosis you must **ask permission to touch** the client. During hypnosis people are in a vulnerable position, lying down with their eyes closed. It could be uncomfortable having their personal space invaded if they are not aware that this may happen. This gives you permission to touch them at any time during hypnosis. If you need to touch them to create an anchor at any other time you already have their permission and they will not feel threatened.

Test yourself

List types of suggestion and tick direct suggestions.

List the four rules governing suggestion.

List three words we use regularly in the language of hypnosis.

Assurance versus Suggestibility

Some books and training courses call assurance procedures 'suggestibility tests.' I prefer the phrase 'assurance procedure' because it makes clear it is for the benefit of the client. I think 'suggestibility test' sounds like you are testing your client. I do not know about you, but I would much rather be assured than tested! So I always tell my client that once I have introduced hypnosis I will then do what is called an assurance procedure, and that it is for their benefit.

I say to them: 'You will be lying there and your eyes will be closed and you will be thinking, "Am I in hypnosis? I can open my eyes if I want to! Am I doing this right?" So I am going to gently lift your arm in the air. I will then ask you to use your imagination, I will ask you to pretend your arm is feeling lighter and as long as you go along with what I am saying you will find that your arm feels very, very light. I will then lift your other arm and suggest that it is feeling very different, it is feeling very heavy. As long as you play you will find that your heavy arm will come down. This is so you know that Yes, you can open your eyes, but you are also open to suggestion. It is because I am trained in the language of the subconscious that I will be able to help you to make the positive changes that you want to achieve your goal.'

When I first qualified, all the books said that if you lift a client's arm and it is not heavy, this is an indication of a lack of depth and you will need to do a deepener. In practice I would say that with about 80% of my clients, when they give me their arm there is no heaviness at all. I deepen them as instructed from my training. However when they come up from hypnosis they say how impressed they are with the 'procedure'!

I thought about this and wondered that although they were not deep, they still found it fascinating! This puzzled me for years until one day I was on holiday watching people in the pool and noticed how easily people when they are relaxed can play, do not analyse everything and just have a good time. This got me thinking about how we Britons are naturally very polite: if there is a queue we will join it, we say please and thank you a lot and we try not to get in people's way. Surely when we are in hypnosis we are still polite and if we hear an instruction that someone is going to lift our arm in the air we would subconsciously assist that person and give them our arm? This was like a light bulb moment for me and I no longer worried if a client gave me their arm. I just assumed that they were naturally helpful and until this day this is what I believe. Just because you are relaxed does not mean that you will suddenly stop being helpful.

It is very important for your client to feel confident and an assurance procedure achieves this if you do it well. I always do an assurance procedure on the first appointment. It gives you as the therapist a good idea of how imaginative your client is. It also benefits the client because they feel assured that they are in hypnosis. More often than not the client will talk more about the assurance procedure than the therapy session! Like anything else it takes practice. Get good at it; keep practicing so you will be confident.

Chapter Four

Deepening the Hypnotic State & IMR – Ideo-Motor Response

As you already know from our staircase example in Chapter One, the state of hypnosis occurs at a stage between wakefulness and sleep. So it would make sense that there are also various depth levels of hypnosis. Some describe these as light, medium and deep states. A deepener technique can be used to deepen the hypnotic state, following the induction and at any other time during hypnosis.

Recognising the trance state / gauging depth

As you gain experience you will come to recognise the tell-tale signs of depth in hypnosis. There are quite a few indicators you can use to gauge whether your client is in hypnosis:

- With the relaxation of hypnosis breathing slows down – watch their chest.
- Individuals swallow as they are slipping into hypnosis or going deeper.
- Fluttering of the eyelids / rapid eye movement.

- The face relaxes into an expressionless appearance, which some call the 'hypnotic mask'.
- Often when a client enters hypnosis they will expel air in a long deep breath, often referred to as the 'hypnotic sigh'.
- Some clients flush and go red in the face, neck or chest.
- During the arm assurance procedure, as a rule if the arm is a dead weight they are deep in hypnosis – but take care, as there are exceptions to the rule and with some clients the arm may be light. I have my own views on this subject, which I will explain at the end of this chapter.

When to use deepeners

Deepeners can be used:

- When you look at a client and you feel they are not deep enough.
- Following Induction – it is a good idea to try out different deepeners as you practise.
- If the client needs to go to the loo during the session just say 'I am going to count from 1 to 3 and then say open your eyes and you will awaken. You will awaken go to the toilet do all the things you need to do, and when you come back in the room you will find that you will be able to relax and drift into a deep relaxation easily ready! 1,2,3 awaken' (note you will need to guide your client to the toilet as they will feel as if they are a little bit drunk) – sit them back down and say, 'Take a nice deep breath, 1, 2, 3' and then use a deepener.

There are many different types of deepener you can use, so I would recommend you ask your trainer for a selection. Try a few and find the ones you like best, also remember that all our clients are different and you may find some deepeners will work better than others depending on the particular client. A particularly useful deepener is the 'eyes open, eyes closed' technique by Dave Elman as it helps you gauge the client's depth of hypnosis.

IMR – Ideomotor Response
What is IMR?
IMR stands for Ideomotor Response: when a client is in hypnosis and deep enough, we ask them to choose a finger that they will use to indicate YES and NO responses.

This skill makes hypnotherapists unique, as it is a technique that bypasses the conscious, analytical mind, allowing us to communicate directly with the subconscious mind.

'The theory is that people may often allow more accurate information to come from the subconscious mind through ideomotor responses than through verbal answers. Since the conscious intellect can filter and/or embellish easily if the person is only in a light or medium trance depth, there is greater likelihood of accuracy when the answer comes more spontaneously from the inner mind.' *Roy Hunter*

Why do we use IMR?
Using IMR you can identify causes and habits that underlie a problem.

It helps you deal with the true causes as opposed to simply treating the symptoms. If you merely treat a symptom, the problem will most likely reoccur. (Here's an analogy – it is no use giving a patient a headache tablet if they have a brain tumour.)

Proficient use of IMR is like any other skill: it needs practice. However, once perfected, it is highly effective and produces results for 99.9% of clients.

Explaining IMR to your client before hypnosis
It is important to briefly explain the use of IMR so your client knows what to expect and how to respond – this sets you up for success.

After you have explained the arm assurance, you can go on to say:

'Then I am going to ask you to choose a finger and lift it in the air, and when you've lifted that finger in the air that is when I sound like a hypnotist because I will say, 'I want your subconscious mind to take control of that finger' and I will go on to ask the subconscious mind lots of questions. That is where I find out what type of therapy to use for you.'

NOTE – Remember to ask the client's age as part of your initial conversation as you will need this information for use with IMR.

Positioning the client's hands

It is important your client's hands are in a comfortable position so they can lift their chosen finger easily. The ideal time to set them up for this is following the arm assurance procedure. As you place their arms and hands back down, you can position them as you wish.

Hands should be positioned:
- Either over the end of the arm of the chair
- Or placed on a cushion with fingers suspended over the edge.

IMR SCRIPT

Here is an IMR script I find works really well.

"While you are resting in this very pleasant way, I want you to notice how it feels just to relax, notice your legs heavy and relaxed, your head comfortably resting in that chair. Now notice your hands as I gently change positions of your hands.

(Place your client's hands in the correct position.)

Now I want you to concentrate all your attention on those hands, and as you do so, I want you to notice everything you can about those hands. Notice the position I have put them in. Whether your hands feel warm or cold. Whether they feel comfortable or not in that position. I want you to notice all of these things.

Now notice your fingers. Whether they are together or apart. Whether they are bent or straight. Whether they feel comfortable or not.

Now notice your fingertips. And as you notice your fingertips, notice just how sensitive they are, because through your very sensitive fingertips you can pick up information about the surface they are resting on. You can tell whether that surface is rough or smooth. Whether it is hard or soft. Whether it is warm or cold. Whether it has a pleasant feel to it or not. All of these things you can pick up through those very sensitive fingertips.

As you notice these things, I want you now to choose just one finger. Any finger you like. And as you do this, just concentrate on that one finger you have chosen. And as you concentrate on it, notice that one finger feels far more sensitive than all the rest. It feels different. It is beginning to feel lighter, much lighter. The more you concentrate on it, the lighter it becomes, feeling as though it wants to float up into the air. As though it is uncomfortable where it is and wants to find comfort by floating up into the air. It is getting lighter and lighter as it begins to float up into the air.

(Keep going until finger begins to lift.)

The higher it floats, the more comfortable it becomes. And it is so comfortable in that raised position, I want you to leave it floating there while I talk to you for a while.

I want the subconscious to keep control of that finger and I want to ask the subconscious mind some questions. If the answer to my question is Yes, I want the subconscious mind to make that finger twitch so I can clearly see, and if the answer to my question is No, I want that finger to stay still and comfortable in the air (*Repeat the last paragraph*)...

I want to thank the subconscious mind for the perfect work it does for (*client's name*)."

Now ask questions, remembering to thank the subconscious for the changes so far and check it understands that your client likes these changes. Then check if it is still necessary to regress to anything. We will be looking at regression fully in Chapter Five.

Questions:

"Subconscious mind, are the events so important we need to revisit them, Yes or No?

Subconscious mind, is it a habit or skill that (*client's name*) has learned, Yes or No?

(*If a habit*) Subconscious mind, is it necessary to look at where (*client's name*) learned this habit, Yes or No?

(*If Yes to look at where this habit comes from*) Subconscious mind, are you willing to show (*client's name*) where this habit came from when I count from 1 – 7, Yes or No?

Do you understand that my role here is to help (*client's name*), Yes or No?

Subconscious mind, are you willing to work with me, Yes or No?"

At this point you may need to ask more questions.

The stages of the process are broken down here:
- Focus attention on hands and then fingers.
- Ask your client to choose a finger.
- Suggest the finger is becoming lighter, as though it wants to float up into the air.

Deepening the Hypnotic State & IMR – Ideo-Motor Response

- Once the finger has risen, tell your client you are going to call out numbers for their age (for example, 39, then going down 38, 37, 36...)
- Explain that if an event connected to their problem took place in any year, their subconscious mind will take control of the finger and make it twitch.
- Make the count. (Watch your client's fingers carefully and note down the ages where a twitch occurs).
- Make the count again, forwards.
- Explain that you are going to ask the subconscious mind some questions and the finger will twitch for Yes, stay still for No.
- Ask questions regarding events, habits or skills.
- Gain agreement from the subconscious that it will help your client with the problem before you both get chance to look at the cause at the next session. (There are a range of NLP techniques you can use at this stage; we will look at one technique shortly to get you started.)
- Ask your client to lower their finger and relax.

NOTE – *Always treat the subconscious with respect. When you have asked all your questions, thank the subconscious mind again for the perfect work it does for your client. Finish like this:*

"Good. Now I want you to let that finger become heavier now. Heavier and heavier, so that it comes back down to rest and joins the other fingers. That's good. Now just relax those fingers and let them feel good. Relax the whole hand, and your arm. If you wish to change position to make yourself more comfortable, then you may do so. Just let your whole arm feel good, comfortable and fine."

Personal view: Achieving goals

I had been practising as a hypnotherapist for about three months and rapidly began to realise that the training I had undertaken was totally inadequate and I was not serving my clients in the best way I could. I began retraining with Lorraine and the difference was unbelievable – I finally had all the tools I needed to help my clients achieve their goals. One of the most profound shifts for me was learning about Ideo Motor Responses and how it enables me to communicate with my clients' subconscious minds, providing a truly client-centred therapy, rather than just relying on reading scripts as so many therapists are trained to do. Lorraine is passionate about hypnotherapy and her training is interactive, friendly and fun.

Graham Parish, Petersfield Hypnotherapy

After IMR
Creating new behaviours / alternative choices – NLP technique

We can use an excellent NLP technique at this stage to start facilitating change. You are now starting to help your client make really positive steps, and this gives me such a buzz. It is why I became a hypnotherapist in the first place!

When to use: This technique is useful to help a client change any unwanted behaviour or habit. e.g. drinking too much, snacking between meals, holding tension in neck and shoulders.

Summary: It involves the client 'going inside' and finding the part of them that runs the unwanted behaviour, establishing what it is trying to do for them and then changing this behaviour for three new positive ones to take its place.

As people, we have every resource available to us – to feel happy/sad, hungry/full, confident/not confident etc. We just have to tap into these resources to reprogramme our behaviours. Here is a great script.

CREATING ALTERNATIVE CHOICES
SIX STEPS TO REFRAMING

" I want you now to go inside and find the part of you that helps you **(to snack/eat chocolate/bread…)** and when you have found that part, just let me know… *PAUSE (wait for a response)*.

Deepening the Hypnotic State & IMR – Ideo-Motor Response

Now I want that part to let you know what it is genuinely trying to do for you and when you know, just let me know... *PAUSE.*

Now I want you to go to your higher self and have your higher self produce three new alternative choices that are readily available, practical and sensible for you to use and will help you to achieve your goal **(i.e. to stop smoking or lose weight...)** *PAUSE (continue when you have a response)*. Now a second alternative choice... *PAUSE.* And now a third...

I want you now to go to that part of you that runs the behaviour of helping you to **(snack, binge whatever the client wants to change)** and ask that part if it is willing to take responsibility for these new alternative choices which will help you to achieve your goal, and just let me know... *PAUSE (make sure that the part is willing and then proceed).*

I want you now to run a movie in your mind and in that movie I want you to see yourself going about a normal daily routine. See yourself using your new and alternative choices whenever you need to and just as you see it now, that is how it will be. Run that movie now and just let me know when you have finished... *PAUSE (wait for response).*

Now bring all the parts round the chair of your higher self and ask all the parts are happy working together to help **(your client's name)** achieve your goal..."

PAUSE
Wait for IMR then check that the subconscious is happy with the new alternative choices and that it will help **(your client's name)** *to be in control and achieve their goal. Thank the parts and ask them to all go back knowing that they are working together to help* **(your client's name)** *to achieve their goal. Thank the subconscious and suggest that the finger is feeling comfortable, relaxed and fine.*

The choice of finger and their meanings
You can get useful information about your client from the finger they choose to use during IMR. Here are some definitions, but do keep in mind they are only indications, not set in stone. Remember, my point about client-centred hypnotherapy is that we treat everyone as unique.

INDEX FINGER – Indicates ambition or authority.

MIDDLE FINGER – Indicates taking responsibility or a person who has the ability to take responsibility.

RING FINGER – People who are very much into relationships; they like to be liked, people pleasers.

LITTLE FINGER – Relates to communication. It can also indicate financial difficulties or relate to sex, perhaps abuse, but do not assume.

THUMB – Indicates a 'Jack the Lad', taking-the-mickey kind of person. They tend to be analytical or awkward. You can say, 'Please put your thumb down, I asked you to raise a finger.'

A finger on the left hand is ideal as this links to the right side of the brain, the creative side, but it is most important to allow your client the choice of hand and finger to use.

Trouble shooting – what if the fingers do not respond?
I have explained how proficient use of the IMR needs practice, but once perfected is highly effective and produces results for 99.% of clients. If a finger does not respond there is a reason behind it because the subconscious mind is not analytical: if you ask it for something the subconscious mind will do it.

Reasons why a finger does not respond:

- You may not have explained it clearly to the client before hypnosis – you will need to move on to a script.
- The fingers may not physically be able to lift – check the position of the hand.
- Your client is too deep in hypnosis – they may have fallen asleep.
- Their state is too light and they are not in hypnosis – use a deepener.
- They are just not 'playing'.

Too deep in hypnosis

The best way to deal with this is to 'wake them up'. Say:

'I am going to count from one to three and on the count of three I want you to open your eyes and come back to full awareness. One, getting lighter, two, coming back to full awareness, three, open your eyes, that's lovely. Now close your eyes and just allow yourself to drift at this very nice level. I want you now to just focus on your hands...' (*Move on to your IMR script*).

Just not playing

Try this:

'Now I want you to take a nice, deep breath and relax deeper and deeper in that comfortable feeling of relaxation and in the next moment, when you are ready, you will just allow that finger to rise.'

It does not matter if they consciously lift the finger because the subconscious mind does not know the difference between what is real and what is not; soon the subconscious mind will just take over control of that finger.

Test yourself

Give two reasons why we use IMR.

During IMR does it matter if the client is consciously moving their finger? Explain your answer.

Write down two reasons why the finger may not respond to IMR.

Suggest two ways to deal with a non response to IMR (no finger movement).

Depth does not Matter

I would like to say a little more here about depth, as this is another subject where my view differs from that of conventional teaching. Again, I hope you will make your own mind up and not take everything I say as gospel, but I believe therapists often get too caught up with depth, to the detriment of their clients.

Depth does not matter. What matters is does your client understand what has caused the problem? If so, they can deal with it.

The way we think is mysterious and as we are all individuals, how can we know what depth is for you or for me? Does it matter how deep you are or if you pretend to be hypnotised? Let us think about this. If you pretended long enough that you had a limp and you limped about, you would end up with a real limp even though there was nothing physically wrong with you.

I heard my daughter Rachel once talking to her friends and they asked her what it was like being hypnotised. She said, 'Oh it's easy. You tell my mum stories. Just make them up.' Which I think is wonderful because it is true. We file in pictures and remember in pictures. So you just say the first thing that comes into your mind.

Do not get hooked on depth as long as your client goes along with what you are asking. If they do it long enough they will make the changes they want. Hypnosis cannot make anybody do anything against their will. If they are not prepared to put effort in, they will not make the changes. But if they do make the effort, whether they are pretending to be hypnotised or not, they will make the changes.

A perfect example is when you sit down and watch TV. When there is a really sad part and you cry real tears, are you pretending to be upset or are you really crying? When you get scared watching a horror film are you pretending? You know really it is make-believe and they are acting! However, if you choose to put your conscious analytical mind aside and believe what you are watching, you feel real, not imagined, feelings. When the adverts come on you jump up and make a cup of tea or coffee maybe go to the loo. You sit back down and there you are back into the film or soap. Your mind is that quick. So depth does not matter and the fact is, the more we practise anything, the better at it we become. So the more your client practises, the deeper they will go. Also, the more they trust you and have a rapport with you the deeper, your client will go.

Another thing I hear a lot is about clients 'popping up' out of hypnosis. If you are confident this is great, as you just 'pop' them back in. This is one of the techniques that stage hypnotists use. Every time you bring a client (or in the case of a stage hypnotist, a member of the audience) out of hypnosis and drop them back in, they go deeper.

A big part of my training is practical. I do not show old recordings of therapy but instead get my group working with each other and me working with them. One of my groups were so much fun to train I called them the Laughter Group, and they gave me a fantastic example of 'popping up.'

My trainee Sally was my volunteer. She was in hypnosis and we were dealing with her eating habits. I started to create some new positive choices and asked her subconscious to come up with three new choices, which it did. Then I asked Sally to run a movie in her mind using her new positive choices, which she did. I asked them to work together and I had no response (I always take that as a No). So I asked her subconscious to produce another three alternative choices for Sally to use, and with no warning she opened her eyes, sat up and looked at me. All I did was stay calm and just said, 'Sally. Are you alright?' She said, 'Yes. I started spinning.' I said. 'Okay, just close your eyes. That's right, take a nice deep breath and just allow yourself to drift.' I then did a little deepener and asked the subconscious mind to lift the finger in the air.

I continued, 'Subconscious mind, do you understand that Sally wants to change her eating habits, Yes or No?'
'Yes.'
'Do we need to look at the events. Yes or No?'
'Yes.'
'Is it okay if we deal with it now, Yes or No?'
'Yes.'
'Subconscious will you keep Sally safe, Yes or No?'
'Yes.'

I proceeded to install a safe place and then went into regression. Sally went to two events. First she was a baby crying in her cot and her mum was trying to keep her quiet as the crying annoyed her dad. Well, mum would give Sally a bottle to shut her up. The second event was when she was two or three and she had pneumonia. She could have died and from then on she was told that she must eat to stay healthy. I dealt with this through very positive suggestions.

When she came up out of hypnosis, I looked at the class and my trainee Dave had his mouth open in total disbelief. The group asked Sally what it felt like when she popped up.

She said, 'It was really weird. My mind did not want to take on the alternative choices and I started spinning. It made me dizzy. It felt like I was floating out of my body, so I opened my eyes and just looked at Lorraine. When she asked me if I was okay I was and it is really weird, because you just do what she says and when I closed my eyes I just went straight back into hypnosis and very, very deep. It is because Lorraine is so calm and not stressed that you feel so safe. When we did the regression it was fine and it is true, I do think you have to eat well.' She laughed and said, 'My Dad did find me far too noisy. I am!' Well, she does laugh a lot. Sally is such a lovely character.

Clients will pop up out of hypnosis. When this happens, do not engage in conversation. Our work begins when the client is in hypnosis. Stay calm, just ask, 'Are you okay?' and tell them to close their eyes. Use the IMR. One of the main functions of the subconscious is to protect and keep your client safe. If you ask the subconscious to do this, it will. Proceed with what the subconscious says. Keep your questions simple and polite and you will remain in rapport with the subconscious.

On the Other Hand

I was once working with a client and used to try out different deepening techniques when she was under hypnosis. I would ask her what she thought and she would always say, 'Yes, it was lovely.' After our third appointment I asked again. She looked at me and said, 'Lorraine, I'm really sorry but I haven't got a clue what you do with me. I come into your room, close my eyes and the next thing I hear is you saying, "Number five, eyes open." I just know I feel great. It's as though I have had a wonderful sleep!'

Chapter Five

Regression

The Second Client Session

So far we have covered the whole of the first session with your client: meeting them, finding out what they want to achieve, explaining hypnosis using the finger test, explaining the IMR and the assurance procedure and building a rapport with them.

On the first session most people do not drop very deep into hypnosis. This could be for several different reasons. I think people are curious about what is happening so they want to listen to what you are doing; also, they do not know you yet. Again, many people have seen some sort of stage hypnosis and it looks to the audience as if volunteers are out of control and doing some weird things. You will have been able to reassure your client about this! You will also have delivered some very positive suggestions, given your client a takeaway recording to reinforce the therapy and made their appointment for the second session.

Preparation for the second session

A small amount of preparation for each client's visit is essential because every client is different. As client-centred therapists we choose the right therapy for the client – we do not fit the client to the therapy.

Since your client's first visit you have had chance to assess their notes and:
- You will have an idea if you will be dealing with causes or habits.
- You will have prepared a selection of possible techniques to use.
- You will have prepared a selection of potential scripts to use.

Pre-Induction conversation

Following the review of your notes, you should:
- Ask the client **how they have got on** over the past week. How have they felt? What have they experienced? How was the recording? Take notes.
- Explain that they **may be talking** under hypnosis this time. 'Last time your subconscious said there were things to look at and if there still are, you will be talking.'
- Explain that you will be using the idea of a **'nice place'**. 'If I ask you to go to a nice place, you do of course know that you are in this room at all times. All I am asking is what you are thinking in your head. If you are thinking of a beach, then tell me you are on a beach. If you do not know, tell me you do not know.'
- State, 'It is your **first thought** I am interested in.'

Regression

Regression is the technique of taking your client back to past events under hypnosis to find and deal with the causes of their problem. You can read about my own regression in the Appendix.

Regression is a very powerful experience for your clients if it is done properly. I believe I am unique in the way I use IMR during regression, and I find it amazing that many hypnotherapists appear to be frightened of dealing with causes using regression.

If you facilitate the IMR well and ask the subconscious if you need to look at the cause and it says Yes, then you will need to be able to do this. It does not have to be traumatic. If you are trained to regress straight to the cause it bypasses the trauma of going back through every time the client has practised the problem – there is no need to keep recollection and recall.

The truth is that whatever has caused your client the problem is not so dreadful that it killed them! They are still here today, and very often if we view something through adult eyes we have a better understanding of it.

I was once talking with another therapist who was very anti-regression and I was intrigued by the metaphor she used. She said, 'If a bear stepped on a thorn and it was painful then eventually it was removed and the paw healed over, why ever would you want to go back and open the wound?' Interesting. My answer to this would be that there is a soft spot and if the bear placed his paw in the wrong place it would automatically open the wound! Why not deal with the cause so that it will never reappear again?

Once your client is in hypnosis (following the Induction and deepener if necessary), prepare them for IMR with a shorter script than in your first session, taking them to the stage where their finger rises. Thank the subconscious for the work it has been doing so far with your client and establish if there are events we need to look at in relation to their problem. If there are, we move on to regression. Here is a good outline script to use.

REGRESSION OUTLINE

"Now be comfortable and relaxed. In a few moments I am going to count to seven and while I do so you will make a journey in your mind. I want you to travel from this place to somewhere you would like to be now, some pleasant place. Perhaps a place you have actually been to where all was well with you, or to some place in your imagination that you know you would like to be.

I want you to make this journey in your mind as I count up to seven. Your mind will easily take you back to somewhere very pleasant for you. And on the count of seven you will be there, and be able to talk to me and tell me what you see and what you are doing without breaking your relaxation in any way, and you will be able to speak clearly and well.

So moisten your lips now to help you speak clearly when it is time to. I will begin counting now from one to seven and your subconscious mind will take you to some pleasant place.

1. Let your journey begin.

2. Leaving this place and travelling (to ... *You need to fill in this space.*).

3. Going in safety and security.

4. Well on the way now.

5. Getting closer and closer

6. Now you are almost there.

7. Where are you? (*Ask other questions such as,* 'What are you doing? Is anyone with you?')

Just enjoy this place now and spend a few moments with the peace because I will now count up to seven again and you will make another journey in your mind going back through time and space to a happy event in your life. (*Repeat as above 1 – 7.*)

Come back now to sitting in the chair in my room. Comfortable and relaxed. I want you to choose one of those places that you have just gone to as your special place. (*Ask your client if they have done this.*)

Protection

Say, 'I want you to take note of the phrase "quickly sleep" because from this time onwards, no matter where you are or what you are thinking or imagining, whenever you hear those words "quickly sleep" you will immediately leave that time and place and return to your special place.'

Repeat.

Continue: 'Good. Now "quickly sleep." (*Test the protection.*)

Now I shall count from one to seven. This time you will go back to (*either age or event*) that led to this problem that you have, so that we may resolve it. If you hear me say the words "quickly sleep" you will leave it immediately and go back to your special place."

Repeat for however many incidents you need to go back to. Always ask whether there are any other events we need to see, Yes or No? 'Do not know' means No. Keep going until you get No. Sometimes you may need to continue on another appointment if you are running short of time.

Tips for successful regression
- The key skill to successful regression is PATIENCE.
- Following the count of seven, PAUSE for 5-6 seconds before asking, 'Where are you?' Then wait. The client needs time.
- If they say, 'Do not know,' ask:
  - Are you inside or outside?
  - Is it light or dark?
  - If you did know, where would you be?

- If they say, 'Nowhere,' ask:
  - If you were somewhere, where would it be?
- You just need to get one word, then you are off; the minute they have a word they will tell you a story.
- You do not need all the details of what is happening. Your client will usually tell you when they come up out of hypnosis.

When you are using regression, remember your client is in hypnosis. When you are in hypnosis you are very relaxed and can find it very difficult to talk. Your client is also processing far more than they are saying.

If you do not get a response, do not worry. You are new at this so simply move on and deliver a script. This will come with practice.

What to do once you get a response
When you do get a response the next most important questions are:

- Do you understand where you are?
- Is this where it all began, Yes or No?

If they say 'No', keep an eye on their finger: it may twitch.

NOTE – You must get a 'Yes', otherwise you will need to allow the client to let this event go and then continue with another regression. In my experience it almost always takes three regressions before you get a 'Yes.'

If the client says, 'Do not know' or, 'I am not sure,' say:
'Okay, take a nice deep breath, 1,2,3, and let all that go.'

Second Regression
Then move on to a second regression, saying:

'I am now going to count from one to seven again and this time I want the subconscious mind to take you back to the event we need to see so that we may resolve it.' Repeat the count and questions.

If the answer is still 'No' or 'Do not know,' get them to let the event go and move on to the third regression.

Third Regression
State:
'I want to thank the subconscious for bringing forward the event (*summarise event*), but this time I want you to go back to the event that you need to see.'

On this third time almost every single client gets there and give you a 'Yes.'

Why does it generally take three regressions? Because:
- Your client is processing so much information it often takes a while to get there.
- You generally find the same person or a similar event comes up time and time again, but slightly differently, until eventually they have a light-bulb moment.

When regression 'doesn't work'
There are many ideas as to why a client does not regress. One very popular with hypnotherapists is that the client is resisting or blocking. Another is that the subconscious is stopping the client from remembering. Personally, I think these are wrong. I believe that we remember the most traumatic things in our lives and we tend to let the good things pass by. The truth is that no matter how traumatic something is, we lived through it and sometimes if we view something through adult eyes we understand it better and once we have dealt with it we can move forward with our lives.

From my experience I have several ideas about why a client cannot get a picture even though the IMR has indicated it is necessary.

I tried to regress one client over about three sessions. His subconscious said he needed to regress and I would go ahead and count to seven and say, 'Where are you?' His reply was always, 'Nowhere!' When he came up out of hypnosis and we would chat, he would say he was feeling angry or sometimes upset. I explained that that was what I needed him to tell me when he was in hypnosis, but he never did. I used scripts with him and he did make some changes, which is all that matters. I do not think he was blocking, I just feel he was not ready to make the changes. Hopefully someday he will be.

Some clients when they are in regression will see colours and have feelings. When this happens, I ask about the colours. For example, one client said, 'It's black.'
I said, 'Where is it black?'
She said, 'In my head.'
'What shape is it?'
'Square like a block.'
'What is blocking it?'
'I do not know!'
I asked her to change the colour. She changed it to grey and said it felt better. I checked if it had gone and she said No.
I asked what it needed and she said, 'Blue.'
I asked, 'Where is blue?'
She pointed to her stomach so we moved the blue up to the black. She was happy. She felt a weight had been lifted.

As therapists, we do have to be able to think outside the box to deal with what comes up. No two clients are the same and most of them have not read the textbooks to know how to perform.

Finally, if you look for a resistant client you will find one. We always find what we look for. I look for ways to help and find a way to deal with what comes up. I try not to lead or suggest, I just keep quiet and use Action Questions (see Chapter Seven).

Distance feelings

At times during regression a client may get upset and say they cannot go to, or stay in the event. There are two techniques you can use to help your client distance their feelings from this situation they do not want to visit.

TV Screen Technique
1. Say to your client, 'Quickly sleep'.

2. Ask them if they would revisit the event as if watching a movie.

3. When they have agreed, describe the following situation. 'I want you to imagine you are at home, comfortable and relaxed, and you are watching the TV, comfortable and relaxed.' Confirm that they are there then proceed.

4. 'In a moment a film will start of the event, you are safe and at home. And as you watch the screen I want you to describe what is happening.' Wait for their response.

Remembering the Event (Preferred Method)
1. Say to your client, 'Quickly sleep'.

2. Ask them, 'Is that the event from where it all began, Yes or No? (If 'No', move on to next regression.)

3. Ask, 'Do you remember the event, Yes or No?'

4. Continue with, 'Was there anyone with you? How old were you? Do you understand why your subconscious showed you this event?'

5. Proceed with Higher Self/Inner Child technique, which I will describe very shortly.

Once you and your client have identified the event that has been the cause of the problem we need to deal with it, they will then be able to move on and heal. We are going to take a look at two techniques:
- Gestalt or Cutting Negative Ties
- Inner Child

NOTE – It is very important that you are trained on regression before using these techniques.

Gestalt technique
We use the Gestalt technique when another person has been involved in the event, creating a negative influence.

Depending on the questions you have used and your client's responses, you may or may not have some background information. If not, it does not matter, because to move on to the Gestalt technique you will just need to ask:
- 'Do you need to cut negative ties with anyone?' (If the answer is 'No' you will move on to the next technique).
- If 'Yes', ask: 'Who do you need to cut negative ties with?'

GESTALT SCRIPT
Say to your client:

" See yourself in a circle of light. A very safe circle of light surrounding you. A place where you are at ease and feel safe.

A little way from you, see another circle of light and in that circle is... **(he/she/them or it could be feelings).** They are also very safe.

Coming from your circle and attaching itself to the other circle is a cord, a rope of light. So the two circles are attached by a rope of light.

Now you are going to speak to... and tell them whatever you need to say, or ask any questions you may need to ask. Remember you are safe and they are listening. So take your time. Either speak out loud or say it to yourself. But when you are finished just let me know.

.... *WAIT. WHEN THEY ARE FINISHED, continue:*

Now on the count of three, I want you to switch and be... **(them).** They heard you, now you are going to be them and hear what you think they would say in reply.

1....2....3.......What do they reply?

.... *WHEN THEY ARE FINISHED, continue:*

Switch now and be yourself. Do you have anything else to say to them? If so, listen again to the dialogue, and again be the other person.

Keep going until your client has finished, then say:

Are you now ready to cut the negative ties that bind you to...? *(If 'No', then you have to find out why they are not willing to cut these ties that are so negative).*

If 'Yes', say:

I want you to see a pair of scissors (or sword) of light in your hand, and when I tell you to I want you to take a deep breath and as I count to 3 I want you to cut that tie and see... disappear in any way you wish. Letting them go with love and light (*if appropriate*).

Take a nice deep breath, 1, 2, 3 and cut."

NOTE – Your client may need to switch a number of times to complete their conversation, so make sure you check they are finished.

Do emphasise the importance of getting them to take a deep breath when they cut the ties. We store things in our solar plexus so taking a deep breath really helps us let the issue go.

Inner Child / Higher Self

Our next technique is called Inner Child / Higher Self. We use this because we all have an inner child and it is important for that child to feel safe.

Pace is crucial here. It is important that you go slowly with this, allowing the client sufficient time to visualise and act on your instructions. Practise will be a huge help.

INNER CHILD / HIGHER SELF SCRIPT

Use this when you have found out the time/event when the problem began. Start by saying:

"I want you now as the adult that you are to go back to that time/event and see that little girl/boy. Can you see her/him? (*Wait for a 'Yes'.*)

I want you to go over to him/her and look at him/her tell her/him that everything is going to be fine. Say appropriate things and take your time. For example:

Tell him/her that you are sorry, tell him/her that they will never be alone again, tell them how glad you are that they were born and what a beautiful little girl/boy they are.

Tell him/her that you are going to take them away and they never need return to this place and have these feelings ever again.

Now take him/her by the hand and walk them away, find yourself and that little girl/boy on a path, maybe a path of your life. The sun is shining down on you both. What does that little girl/boy want to do? (*Wait for an answer. If your client says they do not know then suggest,* 'Walk? Play? Hold your hand? Run?')

Fine.

PAUSE.

Now look up and see coming towards you a very special person. Some people call this person their higher self, their God-like self, their inner self. It doesn't matter what you call this person, they are there for you and the child. (*WAIT*) Can you see your higher self coming towards you? *If 'No', say:*

Encourage it with maybe a light, a feeling, an older version of yourself.

When your client sees or feels something, continue:

Now see the child run into those arms and just feel the love, safety and security that passes between them.

This is the homecoming for the child.

Now you too go into those arms.

This is the perfect family. That fun-loving beautiful child, you the wonderful adult and that very special person.

Now see the child grow smaller and smaller until you can pick her/him up and place her/him in your heart where she/he will always be safe, secure and happy. Where he/she can play and be and do whatever he/she wishes. Have you done that? Good."

NOTE – You may need to cut ties with the person or persons who caused the problem, as I explained above.

Concluding the session

Once you have finished going through the inner child technique, you need to ask your client:

'Is there anything else we need to look at, Yes or No?'

If NO – say:
'Subconscious mind, I want you to just lift that finger back in the air again.
Then ask:
'Subconscious mind, are you happy now to let (**your client's name**) (*describe successful outcome, such as falling asleep easily*), Yes or No?'

If YES – thank the subconscious mind for the perfect work they have done with your client.

If the answer is No or there are other events to look at, say:
'Is it okay if we deal with this next time as we are running short of time? Will you help (**your client's name**) to (*describe successful outcome*) in the meantime?'

At the next appointment you would check progress (continue with investigating any events if necessary) and if your client is moving forward you will then complete the basic structure with the first reprogramming therapy, as I explain in Chapter Eight.

Test yourself

If regression is required what must you do prior to regression?

If during regression a client becomes too upset to remain in the event what techniques would you use to proceed? Name two.

What techniques can you use immediately following regression? Name two.

What would you say if during regression the client says, 'Do not know' to the question, 'Where are you?' during regression? Provide two examples.

Thinking Outside the Box

When Cathy first came to me, she wanted to feel more confident in herself. Even though she was overweight it did not really bother her at that time, she just wanted to feel confident. Cathy and I worked together for a long time (she has said she will be coming forever because she has a fear of abandonment) and I feel really privileged to watch her change. She is such a character and lovely lady.

I want to describe one of her regressions as an example that as a therapist you do need to be able to work outside the box to deal with what comes up.

The subconscious had said that Cathy needed to look at something when she was aged '0'. This does come up sometimes and it has some profound experiences.

I installed a safe place, then proceeded with, 'I am now going to count from one to seven and this time your subconscious will take you back to the event you need to see so that we can resolve your problem. One, let your journey begin. Two, leaving this place and getting smaller and smaller... and on to seven.'

At this point it is very important to wait... I usually count anything from ten seconds to a minute before I proceed with, 'Where are you?'

Silence.

Me: Are you inside or out?

Cathy: I do not know!

Pause.

Is it dark or daylight?

I do not know!

What are you seeing?

I feel dark! I think I am being born!!

What is happening?

I feel as if I am leaving the light and I am dark! I have felt this all my life, that I am dark.

Take a nice deep breath and let all of that go, ready 1,2,3.

Cathy took a nice breath.

Quickly sleep. Are you in your safe place?

Yes.

Do you understand why your subconscious showed you this?

Yes.

I want you now to see yourself in a nice safe circle of light where you feel safe. Have you done that?

Cathy nodded.

Now I want you to see all that dark and light in another circle and that circle is also safe and coming from that circle you can see a cord of light attaching itself to your circle. Have you done that?

Another nod from Cathy.

In a moment I am going to ask you to talk to that dark and light, I want you to say all that you need to say, ask any questions. Remember, it is listening and you are safe. You can either speak out loud or say it in your mind but when you are finished just let me know. Say what you need to say.

Cathy did it in her mind and then nodded.

In a moment I am going to count from one to three then I will ask you to switch and be the light and dark. It has heard you and I want you to hear what it would say in reply. Switch. What does it reply?

Cathy did it in her mind.

Have you anything else you wish to say, Yes or No?

No.

Are you ready to cut that negative tie that binds you to that dark and light and let it go with a feeling of a sense of relief?

Yes.

I want you to see a sword of light in your hand and in a moment I will count from one to three and ask you to take a deep breath and on the count of three I want you to cut that cord and see it go with a great feeling of release. Ready?

Cathy nodded.

Deep breath, one...two...three... cut. *Pause.* Has it gone?

Yes.

I then proceeded to deliver very positive suggestions, counted Cathy up and had a chat.

Cathy said: 'That is really odd. My dad jokingly says I am one of twins and that I took up all the room in the womb and pushed the twin out. I know he's only joking; my dad is like that. Maybe as I was growing up it had an effect on how I felt. I am going to ask my mum if I was a twin, maybe I was.' Cathy also said she had always felt as though there was something missing, like the light!

When she returned for her next appointment, she felt more confident in herself. She had actually said No when her husband asked her to get him a drink. She had said, 'What is up with your legs? You are quite capable of getting a drink.' Well, Cathy has a very supportive husband and he jokingly said: 'I am going to have a word with Lorraine!'

When you are using regression, go with what your client is thinking and feeling.

The Cat Allergy

I think it is so important to get good training on regression. Because if you can do regression well you can deal with causes and help your client move on in their lives. If you are trained properly using the IMR it will tell you whether or not the client needs to look at what has caused their problem. It is not necessary to trawl through the whole of your client's life. You can go straight to the events where the client first learned that behaviour. We never learn how to do something unless we practise. So what happens quite simply is that when we are young we learn how to respond to certain stimuli.

An example is a client who regressed to a garden when she was two. Her mum and dad were arguing in the kitchen and she was frightened. We did the Inner Child, I proceeded with some very positive suggestions and then counted her up from hypnosis. When she opened her eyes, her eyes were really red and streaming. I asked what was wrong and she replied, 'Have you got a cat in this room?' I hadn't. She said, 'Oh my! There was a cat in the garden, that is how I developed a cat allergy.' What had happened was that when she was a little girl crying in the garden, her subconscious mind was monitoring her environment constantly and there was a cat there. So the next time she saw a cat, the subconscious knew exactly what to do and it produced red, streaming eyes. As far as the subconscious was concerned, the problem was dealt with and every time she saw a cat the subconscious produced this behaviour.

My client no longer has a cat allergy.

Chapter Six

Questioning and Maintaining Rapport

Avoiding Non-leading Questions

It is easy to jump to conclusions and get the wrong end of the stick. It can happen when we are talking to people we think we know very well, such as friends and family. But if we are not careful it can also happen when we are trying to treat clients, and that is dangerous. Yes, of course we want to help people, but you may need to check your enthusiasm, especially in your early days as a hypnotherapist, to make sure you are not making assumptions that will lead you off track.

During hypnosis we ask questions in two different ways:
- Speaking directly to the subconscious, eliciting answers via the IMR 'Yes' or 'No' response.
- During regression and hypnosis, where we require a verbal response from the client.

The way we ask these questions is important as we must not offend either the subconscious or the client, as this can break our rapport and lead to resistance, frustration or even anger, all of which can have lasting effects following hypnosis.

To maintain rapport we should always use non-leading questions and when asking questions where the client responds verbally we should, in the main, use open-ended questions.

Let us take a look at some examples.

Open/closed questions and when to use them

Open questions generally begin with:
- Who
- What
- Where
- When
- How
- *Why – we avoid this question. We will look at why in a moment.*

How do open questions differ to closed questions?
- With open questions you cannot reply with a Yes or No, but must elaborate.

These are the questions that will prompt your client to give a verbal answer when you are helping them to picture an event during regression or looking to gather some basic information.

What is a closed question?
- It can only be answered with a 'Yes' or 'No' response.

Closed questions generally begin with:
- Is
- Can
- Do
- Will
- Are

We use closed questions during IMR when we require a 'Yes' or 'No' response from the subconscious via the finger movement.

The WHY question

I have said the 'why' question should be avoided or at least used sparingly and only if absolutely necessary, and you may be able to work out why. If I asked you, 'Why did you do that?' it could make you feel you had to give an immediate answer and it could create a feeling of guilt.

Example

Scenario – Jack comes home from school covered in mud.
Question – 'Why are you covered in mud?'
Feeling – Jack feels he must answer quickly and may respond with a defensive reply. He feels he is being interrogated.
Alternative Question – 'What has happened?'
Feeling – This question suggests no blame so the answer will not be defensive.

Clearly 'What has happened?' would be a better question to use.

SHOULD – This is another word to avoid. It can be a command word and can also promote feelings of guilt.
    e.g. I should go to the gym.

COULD – This is also best avoided during hypnosis. It is a word that suggests 'choice' and puts your client in control.
    e.g. 'I could eat those chocolate bars.'
    e.g. 'I could give up smoking.'

NOTE – Listening is a skill and you really need to listen to your client so that you can build a rapport. Never sit in judgment and if you feel that you cannot deal with someone, do yourself and your client a favour and do not. It will not be good for you or for them.

Leading and non-leading questions
A similar question can be asked in both a leading and a non-leading way.

Example 1:
    LEADING QUESTION – 'Who is there?'
    NON-LEADING QUESTION – 'Is anybody there?'

What is the danger with the leading question?
- It suggests to your client that there is someone there or that there should be someone there. When in fact they may be on their own.

If you establish a 'Yes' to the question 'Is anybody there?' it is okay to follow with, 'Who is there with you?'

Example 2
    LEADING QUESTION – 'Are you scared?'
    NON-LEADING QUESTION - 'How do you feel?'

What is the danger with the leading question?
- It suggests to your client that they are or should be scared.

If you do find that you have inadvertently lead your client then quickly backtrack, as once you lose rapport it is very difficult to regain their trust.

The danger of leading a client during hypnosis
I think the best way to illustrate the dangers of leading a client under hypnosis is to give you two examples, both from my own experience.

Example 1 – Negative
During regression I related an event where as a two year old I was waiting in a taxi office. The therapist (a teacher of hypnosis) suggested that it was horrible for me to be sitting in a taxi office surrounded by

men, clearly implying it was an uncomfortable situation. The truth for me is that I liked the men and in my experience they always spoilt me. This hypnotherapy experience made me very angry and even now still affects me when I think about it, even though it was successful. A further danger is that it could have actually created a false memory of the event.

There is a clear message here – NEVER ASSUME.
(Because it makes an ASS out of U and ME.)

Example 2 – Positive
I was working with a young man I will call Dave on anger management. During regression he went back to a time when he was two. This is how the regression went:

Therapist – Where are you?

Dave – It's dark, I don't know.

Therapist – Are you inside or outside?

Dave – Inside

Therapist – Do you know where inside?

Dave – I am in a cupboard.

Therapist – What are you doing in the cupboard?

Dave – Don't know.

Therapist – How do you feel?

Dave – Scared.

Therapist – What are you scared of?

Dave – My mum.

Therapist - What happened?

Dave – My mum is leaving again.

Therapist – Is this where all your problems began, Yes or No?

Dave – Yes.

This example could have gone the wrong way had I assumed that the boy was locked in the cupboard.

Tips for questioning during regression

- Always ask short questions during regression as clients are processing lots of information, more than they can relate back with speech. Remember in hypnosis clients find it difficult to talk.
- Never assume.
- Use non-leading questions
- Remember it is okay to take your time formulating questions before you ask them as your client in hypnosis is very much in their own head and will not be concerned with pauses.

Establishing the cause
Getting to the root –
During the count on the first visit we will have established a list of ages where events took place related to the problem.

It is important that with regression we go back to the youngest age and the first events linked to the problem. It is here that the root cause can be found: subsequent ages and events will be examples of where your client practised the habit or skill. Once you have dealt with the cause, you do not need to trawl though the rest, the other events will just slip away. It is like a domino effect, knock one down and the rest follow…

How it works –
As adults we view the world very differently to children, so when your clients regress they can view the event/cause through an adult's eyes, rather than experiencing it as a child. As adults we can rationalise our behaviours and adopt a better outcome, clearing the negative effects of the experience.

The next step – reprogramming

Once you have dealt with the cause the next step is to help your client to reprogramme. This involves a lot of visualisation of situations and practising new positive behaviours confidently and with appropriate reactions. In the next chapters we will look at the tools to do this.

Personal view: De-mystifying hypnotherapy

I was helped by a hypnotherapist more than 20 years ago when I was suffering with M.E. All else had failed but the hypnotherapy worked, and so began my belief in this therapy. Now I work as a beauty therapist and hypnotherapist. Lorraine has completely de-mystified hypnotherapy for me and made me see that it is a completely logical process. Her confidence and belief in the therapy is infectious and I have found the whole experience enlightening. She passes on knowledge with such enthusiasm that learning is never boring. I am now able to help people with many different problems, and feel I now have a better understanding of human beings and what makes us tick.

Debbie Hill, Marmion Beauty Clinic

> **Test yourself**
>
> What words do open questions begin with? (Five words)
>
> What words do closed questions begin with? (Four words)

Chapter Seven

Neuro Linguistic Programming (NLP)

In this chapter we are going to:
- Define and understand what NLP is.
- Discover how it works.
- Look at how it can be used to pick up signals/communication from our client, both verbal and non-verbal.
- Learn some NLP techniques that can be used in hypnotherapy to facilitate change and reprogramme behaviour.

NLP – what is it?
NLP is a set of insights and skills with which you can actively use your mind, emotions and body to run your life more successfully and communicate with other people with 'extra-ordinary' effectiveness. It is backed up by a huge range of mental NLP techniques to enable you to improve how you think, behave and feel – and help others do the same.

Neuro – refers to the mind and body interaction.

Linguistic – refers to the insights into a person's thinking obtained by careful observation of their use of language.

Programming – study of the behaviour patterns or programmes that people use in their daily lives.

Who started it?
It was developed by Richard Bandler and John Grinder under the tutelage of Gregory Bateson during the 1970s. This was based upon earlier work by Virginia Satir and also included work by Milton Erickson.

Understanding the principles of NLP – visual, auditory and kinaesthetic
We all take in information through each of the senses: sight, hearing, touch, taste and smell. We represent this information in our mind as a combination of these sensory systems. However, we all have individual thinking patterns that code and process these experiences in our own way, based on our own subconscious preferences.

Think of 'coffee'. What comes to mind?
- Perhaps a picture. Maybe you imagined coffee cups and a coffee percolator or pot.
- Or maybe you heard the sound of coffee percolating. Or maybe the noise as it was poured into the cups.
- Or perhaps it was more of a feeling. The feel of the coffee cup, the taste of the coffee or the aroma of the coffee as it is brewing.
- Maybe it was a combination of all or some of these different ways of thinking.

These different ways of thinking are:

Visual – You think in pictures. You represent ideas, memory and imagination as mental images.

Auditory – You think in sounds. These sounds could be voices or noises e.g. the sound of coffee percolating.

Feelings – You represent thoughts as feelings, which might be internal emotion or the thought of a physical touch. We also include taste and smell in this category of feelings.

Most of us will have a preference for one of these systems over the others, both in the way we <u>think</u> and in the way we <u>communicate</u>.

Working with NLP – effective client communication

Below are some examples of the speech patterns we use, influenced by our preferences for visual, auditory or kinaesthetic/feeling communication.

Visual is seeing words
Language – I see what you mean. I get the picture. Looks good to me.

Auditory is hearing words
Language – I hear what you are saying. That sounds goods. It rings a bell. That clicks.

Kinaesthetic is feeling words
Language – That feels right. I was moved by what you said. I cannot grasp the point. I catch your drift.

Look out for the words your client tends to use most in their communication, clues to help you understand and adapt to their preferences. You will notice we probably use all types of the visual, auditory and kinaesthetic words... but one type will usually predominate.

If they say, 'I don't see your point,' do not say, 'Let me repeat it.' Instead say, 'Let me show you what I mean.'

If they say, 'What you are suggesting doesn't feel right to me,' do not say, 'Take a different view.' Instead say, 'Let us touch upon the points another way.'

If they say, 'I have tuned you out,' do not say, 'You are insensitive.' Instead say, 'Let us talk it over.'

Practice with people you know and listen to conversations on radio or television to develop your skills. Eventually you will find yourself doing it automatically.

Personal view: NLP made simple

Lorraine has given me an understanding of what I am doing so I feel confident to take clients into hypnosis. Her way of teaching is down to earth, relaxed, uncomplicated and extremely effective. Previously I had found NLP confusing and complicated – Lorraine made NLP uncomplicated and simple to apply.

Sandy Wilks, Hypnotherapist

Picking up non-verbal signals

A clue to the way you think is given in the way you move your eyes. If a teacher ever said to you, 'You will not find the answer on the ceiling' they might have been wrong! Our eye movements are usually organised as follows:

Visual – we look up to access pictures. The **left** side is recalling the actual event, the **right** side using the imagination.

Audio – eye movements from side to side accessing internal voices e.g. Did I hear that right? Should I do that? No? Yes?

Kinaesthetic – feeling our emotions. If you notice your client looking down when they mention their mum, there's likely to be some work to do there.

Visual/Audio/Kinaesthetic
Model of learning and information processing

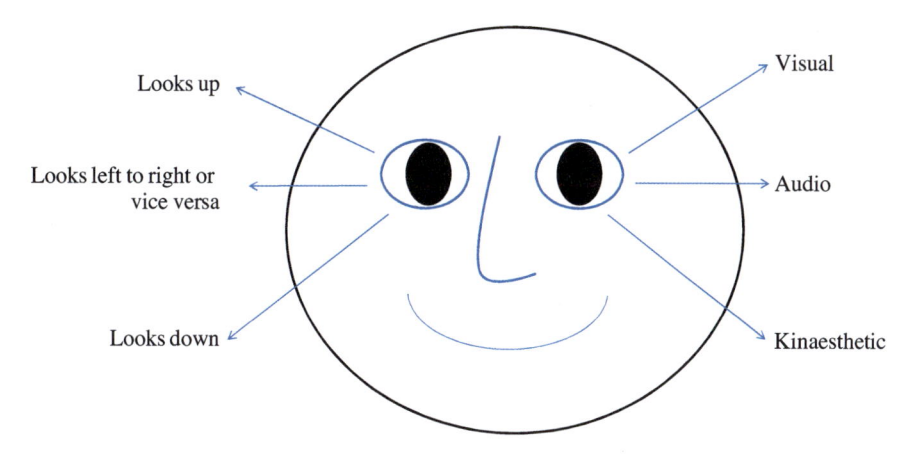

- Looks up → Visual
- Looks left to right or vice versa → Audio
- Looks down → Kinaesthetic

Anchors

An anchor is a stimulus that is linked to and triggers a response. Anchors access an emotional state but we often do not notice them. They can be naturally occurring and result from a previous experience or deliberately created. Examples might be:
- A photograph
- A favourite song
- The smell of freshly cut grass

A person may consciously choose to establish and re-trigger these associations for themselves. You can use anchors to recreate a state and they can be a very useful tool for establishing and reactivating the mental processes associated with many of the changes we help our clients with. For example, a remembered picture may become an anchor for a particular internal feeling and a touch on the leg may become an anchor for a visual fantasy.

NLP techniques
We can use the following techniques in hypnotherapy:
- Pain control
- Rewriting history
- Creating new behaviours
- Timeline
- Swish

Pain control
When to use – This is a very useful technique to help a client take control of pain.

Summary – It involves visualising the pain as a shape and colour and changing its appearance, size and position.

Ask your client to go inside and describe the pain using the following ideas:
Ask how it feels i.e. thudding, constant pain.
Ask where it is in the body.
When you establish where it is, you can find out:
What shape is it?
What colour is it?
Ask your client to change the shape. How does it feel that shape?
Ask your client to change the colour. How does it feel that colour?
Change the shape and colour until it becomes more comfortable.
Ask your client to move it about their body.
Ask your client to make it smaller, or bigger.
You can ask your client to move it to their hand and pop it out.
Ask what they want to do with it.

You can ask them to imagine a dial with numbers on it, from one to five. Five is the most painful it gets, one is no pain. Turn the dial up and down.

When you are helping clients with pain management, do always confirm that they have been checked by a doctor. Pain can be the mind telling your client they have a tumour or something else serious that needs medical attention.

Treating headaches following hypnosis

Sometimes a client may complain of a headache when they come out of hypnosis. Tell them, 'We can take that headache away.' Then use the pain control technique.

Note on treating bereavement

Just a word of caution. If a loved one has passed away recently, it should be more than two years before you intercede. There is a grieving cycle that everyone has to go through: shock followed by grief, anger then sadness, then finally comes acceptance. It is not always in that order, and everyone moves at their own pace. If you feel it is appropriate you can deliver a bereavement script turning death on its head. There may be more work needed, but it should be a good starting point.

Rewriting history

When to use – This technique is useful in dealing with fears or phobias. It can also be used to change our way of thinking about any unpleasant past experiences.

Summary – It involves running a movie in your mind, whilst focusing on all of your senses.

Before taking the client into hypnosis establish that they can picture the situation. If you are dealing with a fear of spiders, for example, check they can remember the last time they saw a spider and have a clear picture of it in their mind.

Induce hypnosis then continue:

" I want you now to imagine yourself walking into a cinema (*check they are in the cinema*). I want you to find somewhere comfortable to sit down and notice that the cinema is empty and as you sit down you look up and see a still black and white picture (*insert the situation i.e. the last time you saw a spider*) on the screen in front of you (*check they can see it*). I want you now to imagine that you are floating up out of your body into the projection room. As you look down you can see yourself sitting in the cinema and out in front of you is the still black and white picture.

In a moment I am going to ask you to run that film in your mind in full colour, normal speed, hearing what you hear, seeing what you see and feeling what you feel. As you run this film in your mind I want you to tell me what is happening, describing what you are hearing, seeing and feeling. Just take all the time you need to run that film. Okay, run that film now... (*Take notes of what they are saying, taking particular care to write down their experience*).

When they have finished, proceed:

Now I want you to run that film backwards really fast...

WAIT.

Have you done that? Now blank that screen.
Now run that film again in full colour speed, hearing what you hear, seeing what you see and feeling what you feel and as you run this film in your mind I want you to tell me what is happening, describing what you are hearing, seeing and feeling. Just take all the time you need to run that film. Okay, run that film again now...

(*Take notes of what they are saying and notice if there are any changes*).

Now I want you to run that film backwards really fast...

WAIT.

Have you done that? Now blank that screen.

Now I want you to run that film forwards again, but this time I want you to add circus music to it. You can make the sounds. You can add funny pictures. Add, for example, pink boots on the spider." *Be creative.*

Keep going until your client experiences change and all the non-verbals match your client's statement. This could take up to about five re-runs.

Example. For years Steph was troubled and upset by the belief that her father thought she was a dreadful cook. (She is actually a great cook.) So I used the rewriting history technique to help her with this.

Steph kept playing an image in her mind over and over again. She was 23 and her dad had come to stay. She cooked lovely dinners full of herbs and spices. After a week she went to her mother in law's who served steamed fish, mashed potatoes and peas. Steph's father said it was the best dinner he had eaten all week. Once Steph had experienced this technique, she said, 'Oh My God!' She realised that she was the one who liked the spicy food and her father actually liked plain food. This instant solution was a flashbulb moment for Steph. Playing the film had made her see the situation from a different perspective.

Creating new behaviours

We looked at how successful this technique can be when we learned about IMR in Chapter Four.

Timeline

When to use – This is a very versatile technique. It can be used to help with fears, driving test nerves, losing weight, in fact in the achievement of any goal.

Summary – This technique uses visualisation. You lead your client to picture themselves in the future achieving their goal. It can also be used in the reverse, where your client goes backwards through the timeline to picture themselves in the past.

Example 'Imagine yourself floating out of your body and just go forward to X weeks' time.'
You can then continue to guide your client on their journey and visualisation or simply say:
'See yourself in the future achieving all that you want to achieve.'

This is also called future pacing. It is a form of mental rehearsal and the nearest you can get to being in the real situation.

How it works

Giving the brain strong positive images of success programmes it to think in those terms, and makes success more likely. Asking your client to experience their desired state or outcome in hypnosis is very powerful. Asking them to run a film in their mind of themselves (dissociated), or seeing themselves in a certain situation (as if in a mirror), will prepare them to experience their outcome mentally before they actually meet it in real life.

Swish

When to use – This is a really useful technique to use in lots of different situations. It really allows you to go with the flow and get creative.

Summary - This technique uses visualisation. You ask the client to bring up a really positive picture of how they would like to be. You then get them to make it brighter and brighter and then turn up the volume.

Next you get them to collapse this picture and bring up the negative picture, turn it black and white and then collapse it on the count of three, with the word 'swish'. They bring up the positive picture as before and again the negative until the negative one fades so much they can no longer see it. The important thing is to be creative, make it fun, spin the picture, the feelings, etc: let your imagination develop the technique. Make them smile. This needs to be fun not serious. People are very quick to learn when it is fun. You are the mediator to help your client choose good feelings, then get them to spin those feelings all around their body.

Action Questions

Finally we are going to take a look at some useful questioning techniques you can use as a therapist both in and out of hypnosis. These techniques have been inspired by NLP concepts. The idea is based on helping people free themselves from the thinking that limits them.

How to help a friend (and yourself) by Michael Colgrass

We all know what it is like to be at a loss for an answer, but have you ever been at a loss for a good question? Here are some suggestions for questions that experts have found to be the best for helping people understand their situation so they can begin to do something about it. They are Action Questions:

What do you want?
What would that do for you?
How would you know when you've got it?
What would you need to do first to get it?
What would you do next?

If they say	You say
I do not know	Guess or make it up
I do not know what I want	What would you want if you did know
I can't, I couldn't	What prevents you
I mustn't, I shouldn't	What would happen if you did/did not?
All or always or never	All? Always? Never?
Everyone, no-one, every time	Everyone? No-one? Every time?
People, it, this	Which people? What exactly? This what?
Touch, hurt, force, drives me crazy	Touch how? Hurt how? Force how? Drives you crazy how?
Makes me happy	Makes you happy how?
Takes care of me	Takes care of you how?
I know you are not going to agree with me, I know what he wants	How do you know?
That teacher thinks I am dumb because whenever I answer a question he smiles	How do you know? You mean every time someone smiles at you they think you are dumb?
I really want that but I have to do this	You mean if you did not do this you'd do that?
Your forcing me to choose	You mean you feel you must make a choice?
Maths scares me	You mean you are scared when you are doing maths?

NLP glossary

You should now have a sound, general understanding of NLP and a selection of really useful techniques to add to your toolkit. The key to success, as always, is practice, practice, practice, give them a go and make NLP work for you and your clients. If you would like to find out more about NLP there is a wealth of reading material available on the subject. NLP techniques are useful in many ways in everyday life as well as in hypnotherapy. Here are a few terms you are likely to come across:

Abreaction: An intense emotional reaction to a past experience. A release of 'out-of-awareness' emotional energy that is deemed in part to be causing the problem (usually distress followed by tears).

Dissociated: When someone is dissociated from an experience, they are watching themselves from the outside – as if they are watching themselves in a film.

Future pacing: Mentally rehearsing and imagining a scenario happening in the future. It is used to test and/or practise a desired outcome.

Kinaesthetic: The feelings and sensations (physical/emotional) of our experiences.

Meta model: An NLP model based upon the language patterns that hide the deeper meaning of what we are saying. By questioning the deletions, distortions and generalisations in our language, deeper meanings can be revealed.

Miracle day: A visualisation that takes the client through a day where their symptoms are no longer with them. It allows them to imagine such possibilities, exciting the mind as to what *can* be.

Test yourself

Why do we need to be careful when using pain control with clients?

Name the three different ways of thinking as defined by NLP.

What is an abreaction in NLP terms?

What is anchoring?

What does kinaesthetic mean?

What is a meta model?

Where do we look to access pictures?

Where do we look to access feeling?

Where do we look to access sound?

Name two NLP techniques we use in hypnosis.

Chapter Eight

The Basic Formula

Reprogramming Therapy

So far we have covered a lot of ground, in fact all of the key stages you need to go through in a client's therapy, so now we are going to take a look at how it all fits together.

We are going to look at how everything we have learned so far can be broken down into 'The Basic Formula' that you can use with every client. Then we will look at visualisation and reprogramming in more detail.

Note I use the word 'formula.' As we know, as client-centred therapists, no two clients are alike – we fit the therapy to the client, not the client to the therapy. The cure does not lie in treating the symptoms but in identifying the causes, facilitating change and reprogramming with positive behaviours and approaches.

The Basic Formula
The Basic Formula can be broken down most simply into three main stages:
1. Hypnotherapy
2. Facilitating change
3. Reprogramming

We use the term stages because we will not know how many appointments will be necessary. It depends on the individual client, their problem and how they respond and progress.
First we will look at the Basic Formula, then visualisation and reprogramming in more detail.

THE BASIC FORMULA

First visit – hypnotherapy
- Build rapport
- Establish your client's problem
- Explain hypnosis
- Explain what will happen during the session (arm assurance, IMR, script)
- Induce hypnosis
- Arm assurance
- IMR
- Clinical hypnosis – deliver script
- Awaken and ensure your client has understood what has taken place
- Make next appointment
- Issue a recoding and explain its role

Next visit – facilitating change
- Review notes
- Gain feedback from your client – establish changes and any changes that need to be looked into

- Explain to your client they may be talking under hypnosis
- Explain that if they do not understand at any time it is okay to ask questions
- Induce hypnosis
- Establish IMR
- Thank subconscious for positive changes
- Check subconscious understands and wants to achieve their goal
- Check if we still have to visit causes
- Is subconscious willing to show client what he/she needs to see?
- When all questions have been asked, bring the finger back down
- Regression (if necessary) – install a safe place and regress
- Gestalt and Inner Child
- Facilitate NLP technique (if required)
- Visualisation – either using a script or creating your own ad-hoc visualisation based on the achievement of your client's goal
- Awaken and ensure your client has understood what has taken place
- Book next appointment / issue recording if appropriate

Subsequent appointment/s – reprogramming

- Review notes
- Gain feedback from client – check progress
- Induce hypnosis
- Establish IMR
- Ask appropriate questions
- Facilitate any therapy needed
- Reprogramming – e.g. confidence programme (three sessions) or further positive visualisation
- Book next appointment (either in one week or a month for final consolidation)

Personal view: Just me and my client

Why did I become a hypnotherapist? I was working in a personnel/training department and came across lots of people who had little or no confidence, which led me to research ways of helping them improve. Hypnotherapy kept cropping up in my research. I trained for two reasons: one, I wanted to make a difference to help people move on in their lives and two, for my own personal development, learning something worthwhile and useful. I like the fact that hypnotherapy is portable, I can do it anywhere, all I need is me and the client. Lorraine is really passionate and upbeat about every aspect of hypnotherapy/NLP so her courses are fun and interesting, with techniques and skills that enhance my work. I highly recommend her!

Kathy Newton, Hypnotherapist

Visualisation

Visualisation is a key component of any therapy. The reason is simple. The subconscious mind relates best to symbols and imagery, so visualising what your clients wants to create or change is key in their achievement of success. Seeing is believing!

Visualisation techniques have in fact been used for thousands of years for emotional and physical healing. By conjuring up positive pictures, visualisation can change emotions that subsequently have a positive effect on your mind or body. Visualisation encourages activity in the right side of the brain – related to creativity and emotions.

If you close your eyes and visualise taking a bite out of a lemon, the chances are that your taste glands will salivate and react as though you have really bitten into a lemon. Similarly, if you visualise yourself running up and down a flight of steps, your heart rate should increase even though you are sitting down and relaxing. These are just two examples of how visualisation techniques can produce real physical changes.

'In hypnosis we alter our internal world. By utilizing our imagination in special ways, we stir feelings and alter behaviour, as well as emotions or

attitudes. When you change how you think, visualise and imagine things to be, your feelings and behaviours begin to change. You not only see what is possible, but your subconscious mind will send up other suggestions for your approval.' Elizabeth Bohorquez, RN, CHt

You can either use:

1. Visualisation scripts – the use of metaphors or stories.

2. Create your own, specific to your client and their goal.

Creating visualisations and reprogramming

Once we have obtained release from the cause of the problem we need to focus on relearning or reprogramming, replacing negative behaviours or attitudes with positive, empowering ones. When you create bespoke visualisations, it is really important to remember to use the language of hypnosis. Key words are:
- Find
- Notice
- More

Remember to always visualise in the positive:
- Weight – see yourself looking in a full-length mirror, notice how toned and slim you are in that perfect size 12.
- Confidence – see yourself in your office and notice how calm you feel as you take two deep breaths. You hear your boss introduce you and you feel even more confident and strong, ready to speak from the heart…

Confidence Reprogramming

With some clients their problem will have resulted in a loss of confidence in some way. In these situations a confidence therapy is recommended to complete the treatment. Once you can see the client has cleared the cause and is making progress you can begin the confidence therapy. During your training course you will ideally be given three scripts: the first two to be delivered in consecutive visits and the final one after a month's break. This allows your client to experience living with the changes for a period of time before you finally check on their progress and consolidate the treatment.

Confidence 1 – Stops your client looking back at past causative events, turning them around to look forward at the future.

Confidence 2 – Takes away the word 'problems' and replaces it with situations.

Confidence 3 – Explains that without realising it we are learning all the time, giving your client the ability to do whatever they want.

You can explain the confidence therapy to the client using an analogy: 'It is like building a house, we have built a good foundation for moving forward, next we'll put the walls on the house and then finally the roof.'

I have worked with people who wanted to stay in abusive relationships, and as that is what they wanted to achieve, I went along with their goals. The funny thing is that after I work with them at achieving this goal and building their confidence, they usually leave the abusive partner and start on the path of an amazing new life. I think this is because using hypnosis deals with causes and finally builds confidence, giving people huge self-worth (although not all hypnosis training teaches you how to regress safely to deal with causes). Once they feel this they want more of the same.

> **Fascinating fact:** Happy people do not just enjoy life, they are likely to live longer, too: a study found those in better moods were 35% less likely to die in the next five years.
> Source: University College London

> **Test yourself**
>
> What are the three main stages of the basic formula?

Hypnotherapy – Natural and Subtle

Hypnosis is very subtle and natural, and often your clients do not notice the changes being made. From my experience everyone has made some changes, no matter how small. So it is very important that you keep good notes: not necessarily reams of writing, but good key words of what your client is doing and what they want to change.

One of my favourite examples is Pippa, who came to me about her weight. Pippa is lovely, she has the most amazing eyes and as you talk to her, her eyes just get bigger and bigger. Anyway at our first session it was clear Pippa had terrible eating habits. She started work at 5pm at Domino's Pizza. Sometimes breakfast would be takeaway leftovers from the night before. She would pick all day on chocolates, crisps whatever was in the cupboards. At lunchtime she would have a sandwich and crisps, then continue picking until she went to work. At work she was surrounded by food and would sometimes have a pizza. On her way home she would stop for a takeaway, usually McDonalds. She lived with her mum Linda who was out at work and did not cook for Pippa.

We talked about her changing her eating habits. If she wanted to snack she would have fruit or yoghurt. She would cook at lunchtime, maybe a stir-fry or pasta. She could have beans on toast before she went to work and a healthy snack when she got home. She would get exercise by taking her little brother to the park and out for walks every day.

I then induced hypnosis and created positive new behaviours and direct and indirect suggestions to reinforce Pippa's new eating habits. I gave her a recording to play and made her next appointment.

A week later she came back and sat in the chair and said, 'Nothing has changed.' She had played her recording everyday.

I asked what she meant. She said she had been picking all the time. I asked what she had been picking? She did not know. She really tried to remember and could not. I asked how many packets of crisps she had had. None. The more we talked, the more she realised that she really had not been eating much at all.

I asked how many takeaways she had had on her way home from work. Her eyes opened really wide and she said, 'None. I've been too tired and went straight to bed.' I asked about exercise. She had taken her brother out every day. When it was raining they walked around Asda. She had bought a yoghurt. I said she had been in Asda with all that chocolate, crisps, sweets and she bought a yoghurt? 'That was what I fancied!'

I laughed. She looked very puzzled.

I said: 'So you've had changes, although it looks like what you haven't achieved is cooking for yourself. You have stopped eating crisps, chocolate and takeaways without even trying. You have been out walking every day and not even thought about that. Today we will work together to help you feel motivated with cooking. What do you think? Pippa agreed.'

This is a perfect example of how natural hypnosis is. The truth is that what I was working with on the first week was picking and exercise, which Pippa had achieved without even noticing it.

I then induced hypnosis and did the regression. As I am an experienced hypnotherapist I do not need to know much of what is happening with my client, I am more interested in them knowing. With Pippa we regressed to the kitchen with her mum and they were looking through the cupboards for something to eat. I dealt with what came up, called the part up that wanted to experiment with cooking and did some direct and indirect suggestion. We made our next appointment.

When Pippa came back she looked much happier in herself. She loved cooking stir-fry and said how easy and quick it was. She told me about all the wonderful food she had been eating, with lots of vegetables. She had even tried lots of salad and she was really happy.

This is why it is important to keep good notes to help your client realise they have changed.

Pippa, unbeknownst to me, had been a member of a slimming club for years (actually Pippa called it a fat club. This is a post-hypnotic suggestion that it is for fat people! I am sure you can work that one out.) Pippa realised that all the years she had been going to fat club she had stayed fat and felt deprived and unhappy. Using hypnosis she had totally changed her eating habits: she had more energy and ate what she wanted, which was healthy food. Pippa said: 'I do not feel deprived. I have decided to stop going and I am going to save the money and come and see you regularly. When Pippa arrived she could not imagine being slim. After three appointments she knew she would be.'

Isn't that fantastic?

Chapter Nine

More Inductions

Writing Scripts

Self-Hypnosis

Hypnosis for Childbirth

This chapter gives you some more powerful tools for working with your clients so that you can adapt your approach with techniques that suit you best and fit your clients' needs.

More Inductions

Most schools and our self-regulation requirements insist that all therapists be trained on several different types of Inductions. While I hope we all dutifully do this, I do feel this is a lot of unnecessary training and a waste of your training time. People are not stupid and I find that if you learn your Induction well (whether it is a progressive relaxation, mental confusion, metronome Induction, rapid Induction or whatever technique you feel confident with) your client will be able to understand it and simply do it. You do not need to be clever and use a different induction with your client every time. Clients like comfort and familiarity so learn an induction that you are comfortable and stick to it. My clients listen to my recording daily and when they come for their appointment some of them are very proud that they knew what I was going to say.

Here are a few more inductions to add to the progressive relaxation I described in Chapter One. You should be able to find one that will feel just right for you:

- **Rapid Induction** This can be quite showy and usually suits the therapist who loves doing things fast. I find it quite scary as it feels as though a chair is being pulled from underneath you. My partner Pete loves rapid Inductions but when he tries to do this to me I automatically stiffen and will not go into hypnosis. See what you think.
- **Mental confusion** I find you have to be quick and alert to do this. As your client experiences dropping very fast, some feel a little out of control. Others find it hard to follow as there is so much thinking involved. Personally I find this type of Induction frustrating, but like I keep saying, do not take my word for something, try it and then make you own mind up!

Rapid Inductions

Rapid Inductions are generally most used by stage hypnotists to drop the subjects into hypnosis really quickly. They can be useful, however, with clients who appear to be overly analytical, overly tired, have any difficulties concentrating or simply have a very fast way of thinking (people who talk very fast). They use a technique called 'pattern interrupt'. The person is expecting one action and you interrupt that normal pattern with something unexpected.

The hand drop instant Induction

1. Instruct your client to press down on your outstretched hand. Say, 'Press on my hand.' While they are pressing down, have them close their eyes, giving them two tasks to focus their attention on. Say, 'Close your eyes.'

2. While your client is pressing down with their eyes closed, suddenly remove your hand. This creates the startle response that lasts for a very short period of time, two seconds at the most. During this 'instant' your client is in a state of high suggestibility. Pull your hand out and your client's hand suddenly falls.

3. Say 'SLEEP!'(in an authoritative tone and delivery, which instantly induces a deep state of hypnosis). However, if this suggestion is not immediately followed by further suggestions for deepening, your client will emerge.

4. Use short and simple suggestions for deepening, such as 'go limp and relaxed, continuing to relax further with every breath. As I gently rock your head, your neck relaxes and that feeling of relaxation moves through your entire body.'

In its shortest form, this is a powerful Induction that can consist of only eight words: 'Press on my hand. Close your eyes. Sleep!'

I suggest you use a deepener following this. e.g. suggest that your client now relax their mind, by counting and relaxing their mind more and more with each number.

Be careful, though. Because this instant induction requires a hand drop that initially startles your client, do not use this technique on someone who is suffering from shoulder, back or neck problems or any client with a history of heart problems.

Tip for introducing this method – start with a traditional induction on the first session and before awakening say,

'The next time we decide to do hypnosis, all I will have to do is drop your hand and say the word, "Sleep," and you will instantly return to this level of hypnosis or deeper. If that is alright with you, just nod your head.'

Mental confusion or analytical Inductions

These techniques work by confusing the mind. As the name suggests, this type of induction is useful with analytical people. Virtually all experienced hypnotists occasionally hear a client say, 'I did not feel hypnotised; I heard every word you said...' More often than not, these words come from the lips of an analytical resister.

While the conscious mind is trying to find the logic in what is being said or done, suggestions are given to the subconscious mind to deepen the state of hypnosis.

Charles Tebbetts, a pioneer of client-centred hypnotherapy, taught two examples of mental confusion.

The first involves instructing the client to close their eyes on even numbers and open them on odd numbers (or vice versa) as the hypnotist counts either forwards or backwards. As you start counting, watch for watering or redness in the whites of the eyes. When either of these begins, start pausing longer when the eyes are closed, and hastening when the eyes should be open. You may add words such as:

> *'It becomes easy to forget, difficult to remember, whether your eyes should be open or closed...and as you remember to forget, or forget to remember, open or closed, odd or even, you just find yourself going deeper into hypnosis...and you can double the hypnosis or triple the trance.'*

At the first sign of hesitation, start skipping some numbers. This helps create more mental confusion.

The other mental confusion technique that Charles taught involves having your *client* count out loud backwards from 100, one number per breath. You may then suggest that your client simply *'relax the numbers right out of your mind.'* Your client's conscious mind gets occupied with saying the numbers verbally while the subconscious is simultaneously hearing hypnotic suggestions.

'As the numbers get smaller, they signal your subconscious or your inner mind to allow you to drift deeper in hypnosis, either gradually or quickly. Soon you can either forget to remember the next number, or remember to forget the one that followed before... or the one that came afterward. And any time you forget a number, or repeat a number, or skip a number, or say two numbers in the same breath, or take two breaths between numbers, you DOUBLE the hypnosis or TRIPLE the trance...' etc.

Once the hypnotic state is achieved it is beneficial to use a 'convincer' such as the arm assurance, to demonstrate to your client that they are in hypnosis.

While mental confusion inductions are great for analytical people, clients with short attention spans may find a mental confusion induction annoying, so it is important to be aware of your clients needs.

Other Inductions
The Water Bucket Induction
Progressive Relaxation
Metronome

THE WATER BUCKET INDUCTION
Taught by Roy Hunter
A mental confusion Induction

Ask your client to extend both hands, palms up, and ask them to imagine holding an empty bucket in one hand, and helium balloons in the other. Also make sure you begin by asking the question, 'Would you like to be hypnotised?' Say:

"Just take a deep breath and close your eyes now and another deep breath and relax. Just IMAGINE that someone begins pouring water into the bucket, while someone else ties several dozen more helium balloons to the other hand.

Choose hypnosis, and you can be totally hypnotised when your hand touches your lap. But for now, just imagine that the water is pouring into your bucket. SEE the water pouring into your bucket. HEAR the water pouring into your bucket. FEEL the bucket getting heavier and heavier. In fact your arm begins to feel like it simply wants to drop right on into your lap so you can drop right on into hypnosis. Or you may feel your light arm getting lighter as the bucket gets heavier.

If your client's arm has reached their lap by now, skip down to the double asterisk (**). Otherwise continue with the following, and skip down to the (**) when the hand drops.

That bucket is one-quarter full now. Every sound you hear just makes that bucket keep getting fuller. You can feel it getting heavier. SEE that water going in the bucket. HEAR it filling up your bucket. It would be SO EASY to simply let your arm drop down into your lap so you can drop on into hypnosis.

Now take a deep breath and relax. As you do, notice your bucket is one-third full now – and you have an increasing desire to let your arm drop. In fact, your arm may be feeling somewhat tired as you try to hold that bucket – which is half full now. And the water just keeps pouring on in!

You feel an increasing desire to just drop that arm... and when you do, you just drop right on into pleasant hypnotic sleep... releasing, relaxing and letting to.

Even if the arm is still up, pay close attention to even the slightest downward movement, keying in on it. Vary your suggestions accordingly, using this script only as a guide.

As you notice your arm beginning to drop, that bucket is almost full now, and it is soooooo heavy!

The instant you start the next statement, touch the palm of your client's hand and speak very authoritatively....

Somebody drops in a rock. SLEEP NOW!
** *In a more soothing voice, continue with the following...*

The balloons are gone. Now just let both arms rest comfortably in your lap. Take a deep breath, and relax even deeper. It feels so relaxing. It is easier and easier to go deeper and deeper relaxed. In fact, every suggestion you accept helps you go deeper and deeper relaxed. Allow your arms to return to their normal weight. They feel totally comfortable, now, completely rested and relaxed."

Continue with deepening.

NOTE – It is important to always remember to restore normality to both arms before proceeding.

Writing scripts

When I teach hypnotherapy one of the many things I train is how to put a script together. When we first start a new job/career, we all need a script and it amazes me when I hear and see other therapists saying things like 'I do not use scripts'. In my opinion, we all use scripts, whether it is making a coffee, driving or walking, for example. We have to learn how to do things in our own unique way.

A well-written script is a valuable tool not only to help you as a therapist but most importantly to help your client.

Remember there are four rules to suggestion:
- Always be positive.
- Use plenty of repetition.
- Visualisation wherever possible.
- Be patient.

With this in mind you begin, writing your scripts.

As an example of positive thoughts, if you have a client who suffers with anxiety, you would not say 'you do not panic', you would say 'you feel calm and relaxed'. The same if you are working with a client who suffers with depression. You would say 'you feel positive, happy and relaxed'.

Think about what your client wants to achieve and focus on the goal.

Secondly, use plenty of repetition; the more we repeat things to ourselves the more likely it will change the way we think and feel.

Visualisation is so important; describe the end goal using phrases like, 'imagine yourself now feeling confident, see yourself walking, talking exactly the way you want to be'. Describe a situation that the client might find him or herself in and describe the situation using seeing, hearing and feeling words. If we can see ourselves being successful, we can achieve it.

Lastly be patient, remember your client has lived with this behaviour over a long time. It will take time for them to learn the new behaviour.

Spend some time thinking about what your client wants to achieve. Start to write the script and come back to it. Before you know it, you will find it so easy to give suggestions and use your creative mind. The more you write your own scripts the more you will develop your own therapy and it will sound so natural.

Here is a great script that can be used in many situations.

THE HEAVY BACKPACK

" As you relax peacefully and calmly, imagine yourself walking down a beautiful country road. To the left of the country road is a field of beautiful flowers of various colours, sizes and shapes. Beyond the flowers is a forest of majestic trees. To the right of the road is a pasture of green grass, at the foot of the pasture is a lake of clear blue water, by the lake of clear blue water are some trees and there is a stream that flows from the hill in front of you. It flows down by the trees, into the lake.

You are carrying a heavy backpack. A very heavy backpack, in fact the backpack contains all of the conscious and subconscious reasons (why you overeat, why you eat fattening foods, why you have trouble controlling your weight/ why you smoke, etc. And can be used for other problems as well.)

You continue walking towards the hill in front of you. After many miles of walking towards the hill the backpack is feeling heavier and heavier but you find inside you the inner strength to continue to walk. You continue walking and getting more and more tired. You reach the base of the hill and you start climbing it.

You are finding it difficult and very steep. Your backpack is getting heavier and heavier. The weight of this pack is becoming limiting and unbearable. You really want to climb this hill but the backpack is stopping you from doing it. Tiring you, limiting you feel the heaviness. You continue to climb but very soon you realises that you can physically go no further. The burden of the backpack is too much. You know the only way that you are going to be able to continue your climb is to let go of the backpack.

I cannot remove the backpack from your back, but you can. You can be free of the heavy backpack. You can choose to free yourself from all the conscious and unconscious problems that are limiting you from finding your true potentials in life.

You have to make a decision. Either you let go of the backpack and all its contents and you continue your climb up the hill or you hold on to the backpack and you will climb no further. You choose. What is your decision?

Attached to each of your fingers is a trigger mechanism that will release the backpack if one of your fingers rise. If you want to be released from the conscious and subconscious reason why you are overweight (or whatever the problem is). One of your fingers will feel very, very light, so light that it will float upwards. When the finger rises, the backpack will automatically fall from your back. Now just allow one of your fingers to rise. It may be the first finger on your right hand or the first finger on your left hand, it could be the second or third, or your little finger, or it could even be the thumb. By lifting a finger, you are symbolically letting go.

That is good. Your first finger of your right hand is floating up. The backpack is gone. You feel free and comfortable. As the heavy weight of the backpack is gone, you feel a greater relief. Now make all the necessary changes within yourself to create the healing that you need in your life. Can you feel this?

Now continue to climb to the top of the hill. You feel so much lighter now. Your body movements are free and you feel refreshed and motivated to continue to walk.

Now at last you reach the summit. You are standing at the top of this hill. As you look below you can see the sun in the afternoon sky. Very soon it will be sunset and you will watch the sun go down and the moon rise. Take a long deep breath and see it before your eyes. You feel so overwhelmed with this beauty and suddenly you start to acknowledge all the things that you need to change your life. You start to realise with so much clarity what you need to do. You now suddenly realise and recognise all the things, all the answers to your questions. It is all so clear now. Talk to yourself. Tell yourself what you need to do. Ask yourself all the questions you need to ask."

Pause.

Awaken.

Self-hypnosis

There are situations where self-hypnosis could be a really useful technique for our clients. These might include:
- Sports success
- Confidence building
- Fear of public speaking/presentations
- Driving test nerves
- Fear of flying
- To reduce stress
- Relaxation
- Sleep
- Positive suggestions
- Habits
- Pain relief
- Anger
- Childbirth

And so the list goes on. Self-hypnosis can be a really useful technique in many situations, helping to give our clients control while they deal with their problem. Self-hypnosis empowers them.

Once you have taught a client self-hypnosis it can also be used to take them into hypnosis in your subsequent sessions with the addition of a deepener.

Before teaching self-hypnosis
1. The client must know what hypnosis feels like, so you will need to have hypnotised them previously.

2. Give the client 'The Rules of Suggestion'.

3. Explain it is important that they focus on positive statements, what they want rather than what they do not want. Provide examples.

4. Discuss with the client what two words they would like to use as their trigger to induce self-hypnosis. Provide some examples e.g. 'calm and relaxed'.

5. Explain what you will be doing:
   - I will take you into hypnosis.
   - Then I will give you your trigger.
   - I will take your arms in the air during the assurance procedure.
   - Then I will count you up out of hypnosis.
   - Then you are going to take yourself into hypnosis successfully.

There are plenty of useful self-hypnosis scripts around, so choose one that suits you.

Childbirth
Using self-hypnosis to reduce pain or fears in childbirth has become increasingly popular.

It has been shown that the use of hypnosis for childbirth can
- Shorten labour.
- Reduce pain.
- Reduce the need for intervention.

- It has also been found that babies born to mothers who have used hypnosis to relax and calm themselves will sleep and feed better.

It is usually just a one-session therapy.
> **Fascinating fact:** The NHS has tested hypnobirthing mental relaxation techniques in studies with hundreds of women.
>
> *Source: BBC News*

There are a number of courses or workshops you can attend if you wish to specialise in this area. I recommend a script provided on a workshop by the Proudfoot School, a very effective and easy-to-use method. The optimum time for a pregnant woman to receive this therapy is:
- After six months. They can then practise using a recording before the birth.
- If they have a history of miscarriage, they can come for treatment as soon as they are pregnant to help induce a calm and relaxed state that will support them through their pregnancy.

You use IMR to check the subconscious understands the mother desires a comfortable pregnancy and a calm, pain-free childbirth. Establish if there is anything we need to look at to help with this – usually this is a No.

Test yourself

Name four situations in which self-hypnosis could be a useful technique to teach your clients.

List four things you should do before teaching a client self-hypnosis.

Chapter Ten

Smoking

There are a couple of ways that you can work to help clients quit smoking. We will take a look at these and then cover my preferred method, focusing on benefits, in detail.

This is a clinical, Direct Suggestion session.

Understanding smoking - When someone first starts smoking, they need to practise to get better. Their body needs to decide if this is a food or poison and so the first cigarette makes them feel dizzy and sick, as their body thinks it is poison. The subconscious then produces chemicals to fight the poison. The next time they have a cigarette their subconscious knows what chemicals to produce so they do not feel dizzy. The subconscious gets very clever and starts to know when they are likely to have their first cigarette, perhaps with the first coffee in the morning. So as the smoker gets up, the subconscious starts to produce the necessary chemicals to fight the poison. Then they have cravings.

Therapists take two distinct approaches:
- Aversion therapy
- Focusing on benefits

Aversion Therapy

This is when the therapist talks about dying, or makes people believe chocolate tastes of slugs. Aversion therapy for smoking tends to go down the route of getting the client to imagine they are in hospital and their family are there watching them die. They are told that smoking is disgusting and sometimes given an association with a horrible taste and smell.

Of course there is a degree of success with aversion therapy, although generally it is short-term: people are not silly, they are aware that smoking is harmful and yet so far this has not stopped them. They know it may in fact be killing them, but they still do it, just as they know chocolate does not really taste of slugs.

There can also be negative effects. I have had clients come to me because the aversion therapy they had elsewhere upset them so much that as soon as they left the hypnotherapist's room they promptly lit up a cigarette because they felt stressed. Every time they lit up they found themselves getting more stressed usually because they were thinking about dying.

Focusing on benefits

This works with the concept, 'What's in it for me?' and involves you and your client focusing on the benefits of quitting, a technique designed to produce long-term better results. Get your client to tell you the benefits they will get e.g. healthier, richer, freedom. Remember to focus on each individual client.

Preparation

You need to establish:
- Their habits – how many they smoke per day/week, as well as their age.
- That they really do want to give up.

It is no use if the client is only there because their partner has forced them to do it. Hypnosis cannot motivate someone to give up smoking. If your client is very motivated you can help. They really need to want to do it for it to work successfully.

Questions
During the consultation use open/action questions, such as:
- Do you want to give up smoking?
- What is motivating you to give up? (Reasons why they have come now)
- How long have you been smoking? How many per day?
- Have you given up before? How?
- What got you started again?
- When do you have your first cigarette? (Change habit/actions)
- What are the benefits of giving up that are important for you?
- What are you going to miss? (Disadvantages)
- What are you going to do instead?
- How are you going to exercise more? (Healthy eating?)
- Also discover their achievements, what they are proud of.

Weight
When a smoker gives up smoking they tend to put on weight. You will need to discuss this with them. Because not only do they eat more, but when they stop smoking their metabolism slows down too. Smoking speeds their metabolism up, every time they light up a cigarette their heart rate increases. Smokers often think that smoking relaxes them when in fact it speeds everything up. The metabolism does return to normal but usually this will take about a year.

Ask your client what they are going to do about this. You might discuss increasing their exercise, maybe by walking. Multivitamin B speeds up metabolism (I always advise clients to go to Holland & Barrett, as the staff are correctly trained and very professional.

Remember that herbs and vitamins are drugs and they will need to take the correct amount for their size and shape). A glass of pineapple juice in the morning can also help with the metabolism.

How many sessions – and what to charge?

I recommend offering smoking therapy as just one session, as this encourages the client to give up straight away. You can also do a two-session therapy; the first appointment would be to deal with giving up smoking and the second to help the client deal with stress. A lot of smokers who have given up for years will go back to it when something stressful happens in their lives. On the second appointment you can teach your client self-hypnosis.

My advice is to charge a higher rate than for your normal therapy. When you are working with smokers, do not be cheap. Smokers spend a lot of money on cigarettes. The more you charge, the higher your success rate. If you charge double your normal fee for your one session, your client will soon still make their money back. It is about value: your client needs to value the therapy as hypnosis is not a magic wand. They must put their own effort in to achieve their goal. If you offer a give-up-smoking session followed by a stress session, you might charge double for the first and your usual fee for the second.

FORMAT OF THE THERAPY

Induce hypnosis.
    Perform the arm assurance test.
    Use a short version of the IMR script. You do not need to count through the ages as usually people start smoking in their teens. Also, the reason they continue to smoke may not have any relation to why they started in the first place.
Ask the following questions:

'Subconscious mind, do you understand that (**your client's name**) has come here today to become a non-smoker? Yes or No?

Is there any reason for (**your client's name**) to continue smoking? Yes or No?

If Yes, ask, 'Will you show (**your client's name**) what they need to see (so they can become a permanent non-smoker)? Yes or No?

Will (**your client's name**) then become a non-smoker? Yes or No?

Note: When you ask the subconscious if it understands that your client has come here today to be a non-smoker, you have got to get a Yes.
*If you get a No, you would then say, 'Subconscious mind, is there any reason for (**your client's name**) to continue smoking, Yes or No?' If the subconscious says Yes, you proceed with, 'Subconscious mind, will you show (**your client's name**) what they need to see so they can become a permanent non-smoker.' You should get a Yes.*

You then proceed to regression. It is not always necessary to install a safe place with smokers. If you feel confident enough, just proceed straight to regression, saying, 'I am going to count from 1 to 7 and on the count of 7 the subconscious will take you to the event you need to see so that you can become a permanent non-smoker.' Deal with what comes up. You may need to use Inner Child and/or Gestalt/Cutting Ties.

Optional: You can then use Creating New Alternative Choices or Swish (seeing themselves as a non-smoker.)

Once you have dealt with what has come up (and used NLP techniques), ask the subconscious mind if your client will now become a permanent non-smoker, Yes or No? If you get a Yes, proceed to a script.
Here's an example: 'Subconscious mind, can you go inside and make all the adjustments necessary for (**your client's name**) to become a permanent non-smoker? And when you have done that, just let me know by moving that finger.'

Deliver a smoking script.

Warning: Do not record the smoking script as you will be giving your therapy away. There are take-away recordings for use with the smoking therapy, so give these away instead.

This method brings a great deal of success. Sometimes clients will come back and if this happens, you will need to assess the situation and deliver the therapy with more conviction.

If you choose to specialise in helping smokers, there are more detailed techniques available. Hampshire School of Hypnotherapy, for example, runs a Parts Therapy CPD course that provides excellent grounding.

KAREN AND THE ASHTRAYS

Karen was an occasional smoker. I mean she really was, she did not need to smoke all day and just enjoyed a cigarette occasionally, maybe four or five cigarettes a day. I do always ask my clients if they have ever given up before and if they have, how and what caused them to take it up again. Karen had given up very successfully with hypnosis but when she became stressed she would go back to smoking again.

I took Karen into hypnosis and asked her to choose a finger and checked the subconscious understood that Karen wanted to be a permanent non-smoker.

I asked if there was any reason for Karen to continue smoking. 'Yes,' was the reply.

I asked, 'Subconscious mind, if we looked at the reason for Karen to continue smoking, will Karen then be able to be a permanent non-smoker?' Yes.

'Will you show Karen what she needs to see?' Yes.

I then proceeded to install a safe place and then counted from one to seven to the event the subconscious said she needed to see. At seven, I asked, 'Where are you?'

Karen replied: In the lounge.

I asked: Is anybody there?

My Granddad

How is this connected to your problem of smoking?

I am playing with my granddad's ashtray and I love the smell of ashtrays.

How old are you?

Five.

Is this where it all began?

Yes.

Do you understand why your subconscious is showing you this?

Yes.

I then proceeded with Inner Child and Gestalt.

I checked with the subconscious that Karen could now be a permanent non-smoker, then proceeded to deliver my smoking script.

I counted Karen up out of hypnosis and we had the after chat. She told me about the ashtrays that used to have a button on and how, when you would push it down the cigarettes and the ash would go into the bottom. She really loved her granddad and oddly enough the smell of ashtrays!

What I think happened with Karen was that whenever she got stressed the subconscious would think, 'I know what Karen likes, the smell of cigarettes', and she would then have the urge to smoke. When actually what she loved was the feeling about her Granddad.

Again, for me this is about keeping things simple and empowering your client to make changes.

Chapter Eleven

Weight Problems

The first and most important point we need to understand about weight problems is that they are psychological in nature. To understand why this is true it will be useful to look at the following four facts. This will help paint a picture of our philosophy and approach to weight problems and their treatment.

1. Thin people have weight problems too

It is not just heavy people who have a weight problem; in fact many thin people do too.
- Many 'thin' people only remain this way because they constantly watch what they eat, are permanently on a diet and are fighting the temptation to put on weight.
- Anorexics have a weight problem too, but in their case the problem is too little weight rather than too much.

So it is clear that weight problems are highly individual and impossible to treat without establishing and treating the real causes.

2. Diets do not work

We are a diet-oriented population. The general premise is that a person is overweight because they over-eat, so they are put on a diet to eat less. They may lose weight in the short term but put it all back on again when they stop the diet; this leads to yet another diet and the 'Yo Yo' effect. Diets do not work.

Diets make people unhappy as they struggle with the concept of 'right' and 'wrong' foods, constantly depriving themselves. This concept goes against what hypnotherapists believe in and the basic philosophy on which hypnotherapy is built.

As hypnotherapists we believe that the subconscious is responsible for the maintenance and operation of the physical body, producing chemicals to do certain jobs, chemicals that affect both our psychological and physiological status. The production of these chemicals is dependent on the raw materials extracted from a selection of food and drink, so by cutting out 'wrong' foods we could be depriving the subconscious of the basic tools it needs to operate. This could then lead to other problems. For this reason diets go against the philosophy of the subconscious and hypnotherapy.

And as diets do not work, there must be another way. It is this: treating weight as a psychological problem and dealing with it using the basic formula.

3. How thin people think

To help us understand weight as a psychological problem it is useful to consider how 'thin' people, without a weight problem, think about food.

They do the following:
- They only eat when hungry.
- They eat what they want to eat. They do not have 'wrong' or 'right' foods.
- They savour each mouthful, conscious of what they are eating and enjoying the taste.
- When they have had enough and are no longer hungry they stop eating, leaving food on the plate if they have had their fill.

Once any causes have been identified and cleared, hypnotherapy can help a client think in this healthy way about food.

4. Listening to your body, the benefits and changes

When we remove the concept of right and wrong foods a client may at first be concerned, because it is contrary to the concept of dieting and deprivation so ingrained in our society. In its place we can explain the importance of learning to listen to our body, more specifically in fact our subconscious, as it tells us what foods we need to eat.

e.g. A pregnant woman's fancies or cravings.

It is normal to fancy certain foods; it is our body's way of telling us what it needs. When we follow our instincts we feel good, if we do not, they nag at us and we feel miserable, often the reason why most people on diets feel unhappy.

Different chemicals are needed to make us happy or unhappy, so when a client's thinking changes, so too will the signals from their body. As a result, tastes and fancies alter in accordance with our positive way of thinking.

What is more, less effort is required in being happy than in being unhappy so less fuel is required to drive this positive state – so the quantity of food needed will reduce.

> **Fascinating fact:** In the UK an estimated 60.8 per cent of adults and 31.1 per cent of children are overweight. According to figures from 2009, almost a quarter of adults (22 per cent of men and 24 per cent of women) in England were classified as obese (BMI 30kg/m^2 or over).
>
> *Source: BBC*

Building a therapy
Now we understand the background and our philosophy of dealing with weight problems we can move on to looking at the structure of the therapy itself.

First visit
Initial consultation
1. Establish your client's current eating and exercise habits.
    e.g. Ask them to describe a typical day of what and how they eat.
    e.g. Find out what they do to get moving or what exercise they do during a normal week?

2. Listen and take notes. It is likely they may not reveal the whole truth about their eating habits, so you may need to delve a bit deeper.
    e.g. Ask what else do you do or eat that may have contributed to your weight gain?
    This may reveal snacking, large portions, 'can't say no', etc.

3. Establish their goals: eating, exercise, and what they want as an end result. Ask:
    e.g. How would you like to eat?
    e.g. How would you like to exercise?
    e.g. What size/weight would you like to be?
    e.g. Can you picture how you would like to look?
Make sure their goal is achievable and they can picture how they would like to look.

5. Summarise and ensure you have identified any changes they need to make.
    e.g. Snacking, sweet tooth, binge eating, comfort eating.
Ensure they are happy with any changes to eating or exercise habits you have discussed and if they followed the plan they believe they would lose weight.

Next steps
- Follow your usual preamble: explain hypnosis and what will happen.
- Induce hypnosis.
- Arm assurance.
- IMR – check subconscious understands your client wants to lose weight.
- IMR – find out if causes need to be dealt with, habits, etc.
- IMR – count through ages.
- Create new behaviours and positive alternative choices.
- Deliver a weight-loss script from the many that are available.
- Give your client a recording to take away to reinforce the therapy.

Scripts and aversion therapy

Most popular weight-loss scripts take a very positive, health and wellbeing-focussed approach to weight loss. Others take a different approach based on aversion therapy. Aversion therapy provides negative, repulsive images (sometimes frightening) designed to put you off or 'avert' you from the behaviour.

In my view it provides only temporary effects, as I outlined in Chapter Ten on smoking. People are not stupid, they know the 'aversion images' are not true: there are not really snakes in the biscuit tin. If you do decide to use aversion therapy on occasion, make sure the images you provide cannot be validated – that your client cannot check it out. For example if you talked about how our food is made in the factories. How we do not really know what happens to it before it arrives at the supermarket do we really know how food is prepared?

On the whole it is preferable to take the positive approach because people are geared to learn, find and grow things.

Second visit – facilitating change

- Following review of your notes, ask your client how they have got on and confirm that their new alternative choices are working.
- Explain that in this session you will be looking at causes if necessary and if so they will need to talk during hypnosis.
- Induce hypnosis.
- Use the short version of IMR.
- Check the subconscious is happy with the new behaviours and double check if they need to deal with causes or habits.
- Regression if necessary.
- Gestalt and Inner Child/Higher Self.
- Visualisation.
- Awaken, discuss.
- Make the next appointment.

Subsequent visit

By this appointment you should find your client is making some changes. They will have started listening to their bodies. Sometimes, though, they forget how they were when they first started the therapy so you may have to prompt them by going back to your original notes and referring back to their orignal habits and asking them what has changed.

As long as progress has started you can then begin reprogramming using visualisation of them reaching their goal followed by the confidence therapy I described in Chapter Eight.

Test yourself

What information should you establish during your consultation prior to beginning therapy for weight loss?

Vegetables

When you are working with clients it is very important to spend time finding out how they eat and how they want to eat. I do make sure I point out that I am not a nutritionist, but in my opinion most of us know what we need to do even if for some reason we do not do it.

Jill wanted to lose two stone. She did not eat vegetables because she did not like them. She ate out a lot, ordering only meat and potatoes. We chatted and I asked her if there were any kind of vegetables she would eat and she said she did not mind carrots or peas. There is usually something a client will eat and it is up to us as therapists to find this information out. I also asked her if she would like to eat vegetables and she said she would, so we talked about what vegetables she would like to try. She said maybe broccoli and cauliflower.

Under hypnosis, I asked the subconscious if it understood Jill wanted to lose weight and eat healthily and it agreed. I then did visualisation suggesting she would find herself wanting to taste new food (broccoli) and asked the subconscious mind to bring forward the part of Jill that wanted to achieve this goal and make it bigger and stronger, which it did.

At the next appointment Jill had had a really good week. The evening after our first session she had been out to a Harvester for dinner and went to the salad cart for a bowl of salad to go with her steak and chips, she said she really enjoyed the salad and only ate two chips. 'Not because I was depriving myself, because it was what I wanted,' she said.

We needed to deal with what caused her to have a weight problem and went back to when she was a little girl. She was in a children's home and made to eat everything on her plate. After we had dealt with the cause, we did a lot of visualisation seeing her eating more and more healthy food. Jill went onto lose her two stone and a little more.

She now loves veg and even when she goes out she now take a bag of carrots to snack on!

Richard's Wife

Richard was 74 and needed to lose four stone for his health. He had tried all sorts of diets but never lost more than a few pounds.

When he arrived for his first appointment he asked if his wife could come with him. I personally do not have a problem with someone coming in with my clients and agreed. I collected him at reception and although it is only a short walk to the lift Richard was huffing and puffing.

I took Richard into hypnosis but when I asked the subconscious mind if it understood that Richard wanted to lose weight the answer was a clear No.

I am aware that sometimes the subconscious does not understand so I reworded the question and said, 'Do you understand that Richard has come here today and asked me to help him lose weight?' Yes.

'Are you willing to help Richard lose weight?' No.

'Do you understand my role here is to help and are you willing to work with me?' Yes. 'Will hypnotherapy help Richard lose weight?' No.

I could not get the subconscious to agree!

When you have a scenario like this, there is nothing you can do. I always respect the subconscious and if the subconscious says No after a few attempts at rewording I will go on and use positive suggestion, thanking the subconscious for coming forward and communicating with me. I went on, made a very positive CD (when I work with clients I record the clients sessions live. This does take a lot of practice and as a hypnotherapist you will need to be confident at recording. I would not advise that you do this until you are confident.), and counted Richard up from hypnosis.

When Richard opened his eyes I told him the subconscious had said hypnotherapy would not help but he said it had to and he wanted to proceed. He looked at his wife and said the problem was all the food she fed him. I chatted to his wife, who would cook him a full English breakfast every morning with hash browns, sausages, bacon and toast. Then she would go shopping and bring him back a cake. She would make sandwiches for lunch, then give him another snack in the afternoon and a big evening meal.

He did not need to eat it but he came from the you-must-eat-everything-on-your-plate generation. It was hard-wired. Richard's wife very reluctantly agreed to change his diet. She was adamant she had no unhealthy food at home until Richard pointed out all the hash browns and frozen chips in the freezer. She refused to throw it away, even though it was affecting Richard's health, but agreed to give it to neighbours.

At the next appointment Richard had lost an amazing stone in a week, just by changing his diet. We needed to deal with causes. I have no idea what Richard went back to as he went so deep in hypnosis he talked very little. He did however say that he understood and we went back to the time when he was in the Forces.

Richard had four appointments with me and during that time he went to Cornwall, where he was amazed he did not want his usual fish and chips. I always leave a gap before the last appointment to make sure my clients are happy with their new behaviours. When Richard and his wife arrived for his last appointment and walked from reception to the lift it was incredible – Richard was not huffing and puffing and he had lost three stone. Brilliant. His wife proudly told me she had lost a stone as well. I laughed and said it was buy one, get one free!

Stir-Fry

I have found some women living on their own lose interest in cooking especially when their children have grown up and left home, even though they have cooked for many years and brought up a family on a healthy diet.

Sometimes people are under the impression that processed prepared meals are easier than cooking. Yet when I ask my clients if they would feed such food to their children the answer is often No!

I personally find stir-frys are very easy and quick, you only use one pan and you can add any meat or vegetables as you like. I point out the benefit of eating healthy food and how it tastes so much better. This often helps people living on their own and they tell me about some of the wonderful food they have started cooking.

One client once admitted she already knew all I was saying and it is odd they never work it out for themselves. Sometimes all clients need is a gentle reminder that they have self-worth and this is where we come in!

Chapter Twelve

Fears and Phobias

Driving Test Nerves

Improving Performance

This chapter covers many more of the problems clients will come to you with. By learning simple techniques you will be able not just to treat them, but to transform their lives. How good is that? We will be looking at:
- Fears and phobias
- How they develop
- Levels of fear
- How we treat them
- A technique to 'Take Control'
- Driving test fears or nerves
- Improving performance

Fear – what, how and why

Fear is a basic, natural, human emotion. It is a mechanism designed to protect us and is essential for our survival. Fear stimulates our 'fight or flight' mechanism, which urges us to either proceed with caution or run away.

The physical effects are easy to recognise: higher heart rate, increase in blood pressure and faster, shallower breathing.

Fear is concerned with the future; it is a fear of what might happen, not a fear of what has happened and as a result our imagination plays a big part in fear.

Levels of fear

Fear can be categorised into a number of levels, based on its intensity:

Apprehension – the lowest level of fear, an uneasy feeling.
Example – Going for a job interview.

Anxiety – a greater feeling of concern, the next stage up.
Example – Going to the dentist or airport; exam nerves.

Both apprehension and anxiety are normal expressions of fear, where the body is working as it should, heightening our awareness until the situation has passed and everything returns to its normal state.

Anxiety Reactions – where an individual spends most of their time in high tension, prone to anxiety or panic attacks. This is not a normal, healthy state and is where treatment becomes necessary.
Example – People have real panic attacks, such as about driving, fear of spiders or fear of tunnels.

Phobias – the most extreme form of fear. This is an anxiety condition where the body is permanently on alert in case of exposure to the stimulus, generally linked to past memories, real or imagined.

A fear becomes a phobia when you have to change your lifestyle to manage it.

Sufferers know their fear is irrational but this does not help them. Avoidance of the stimulus can affect their whole lives as they go to great lengths to keep away from it. If the phobia cannot be avoided entirely the sufferer will endure the situation or object with marked distress and significant interference to their social or working life.

Fear and the body's chemical reactions

When a person experiences fear the 'fight or flight' mechanism trips in, stimulated by the autonomic nervous system (ANS). When fear subsides, the ANS goes back to a normal state; however, a person with continuous feelings of fear has an imbalance in the autonomic nervous system. You will learn more about the ANS in Chapter Fifteen.

Fears

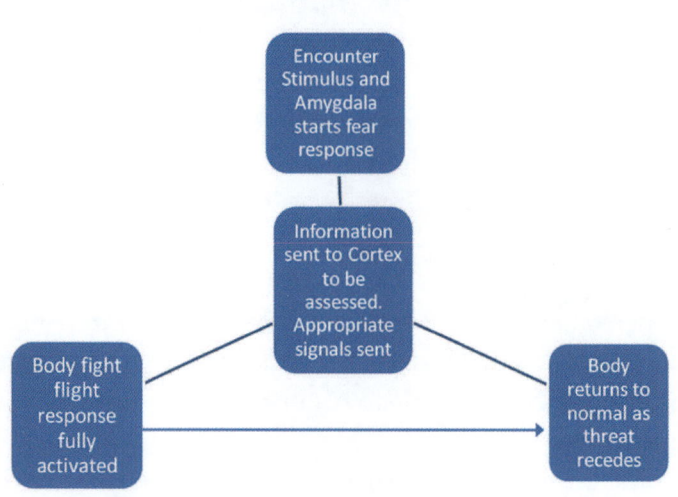

- Encounter Stimulus and Amygdala starts fear response
- Information sent to Cortex to be assessed. Appropriate signals sent
- Body fight flight response fully activated
- Body returns to normal as threat recedes

Phobia

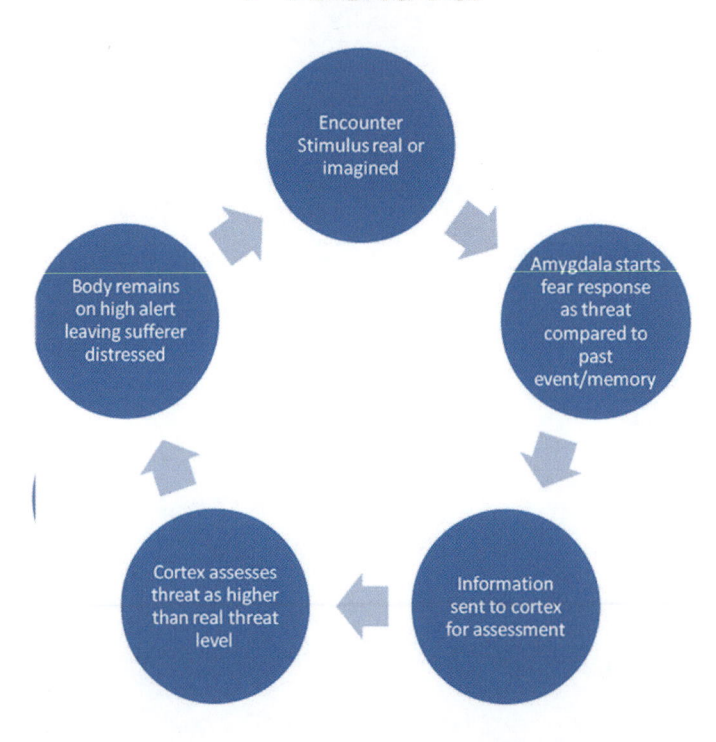

- Encounter Stimulus real or imagined
- Amygdala starts fear response as threat compared to past event/memory
- Information sent to cortex for assessment
- Cortex assesses threat as higher than real threat level
- Body remains on high alert leaving sufferer distressed

Top Ten most commonly reported phobias in the UK

1. Social Phobia – Fear of interacting with other people.
2. Agoraphobia – Fear of open, public spaces.
3. Emetophobia – Fear of vomiting.
4. Erythrophobia – Fear of blushing.
5. Driving Phobia – Fear of driving.
6. Hypochondria – Fear of illness.
7. Aerophobia – Fear of flying.
8. Arachnophobia – Fear of spiders.
9. Zoophobia – Fear of animals.
10. Claustrophobia – Fear of confined spaces.

So it figures that as a hypnotherapist you are likely to come across some of these in the course of your work.

Social Phobia may start off as shyness, which then becomes exaggerated to the point of disrupting your client's life.

Agoraphobia is often associated with panic attacks and sufferers avoid places that spark this panic.

Common Treatments
Drugs
Drugs, such as Beta Blockers, are prescribed by the medical profession. These take away the physical symptoms of fear but they cannot be considered a cure because as soon as the drug is taken away the symptoms return. Drugs can be useful if combined with the technique of systematic desensitisation.

Systematic Desensitisation
This is a technique whereby a psychologist, along with the client, develops a list of activities in relation to the fear; at the start a mildly difficult task, followed by a gradual build-up in intensity, culminating in direct exposure to the fear. Drugs can be used alongside this to reduce the physical aspects of the fear as the client builds their tolerance.

Flooding
The flooding technique involves exposing the client to the fear for at least three hours. The timing is important because it takes the average person three hours to go through all the emotions before they are ready to calm down. Though rather unpleasant it is effective. Both flooding and systematic desensitisation have an 80% success rate.

Treating fears with hypnotherapy
To treat fears we follow our usual Basic Formula. Of course our advantage, and a key area of focus, is establishing the cause through a thorough investigation, then facilitating change followed by reprogramming.

NOTE – If a client is taking drugs they should never be advised to stop taking them suddenly. Once their treatment is well underway they can cut down on them gradually.

Hypnosis and desensitisation

Desensitisation can also be used in conjunction with hypnosis. Rather than working with the conscious mind we deal with the subconscious mind and rehearse the activities during hypnosis before tackling them for real.

'Taking Control' technique

This technique provides your client with a tool they can use whenever they begin to feel anxious or stressed if faced with a particular situation.

When to use it

It is useful in the following situations:
- When your client has a particular obstacle they want to overcome.
- For people who have panic attacks or experience anxiety in any situation.

Examples: fear of spiders, heights, flying, crowds, driving anxieties.

How to use the technique

1. Prior to hypnosis, once the client has explained their problem, establish what they want to achieve.
   Example: This technique was used with a woman with social phobia; she felt unable to go out where there were other people. When asked what she wanted to achieve she said she wanted to be able to go shopping at normal times of the day (rather than at night when the shops were empty).

2. Establish prior to hypnosis a typical example of what they experience in the situation. You will need to use this information during the facilitation of the technique.

3. Prior to hypnosis explain to the client that you will be teaching them a technique to deal with their fear and that

to do this they will need to practise. Explain that every time they experience fear/anxiety during the session that they will need to signal to you by raising their arm, then take a deep breath and say 3–2–1 to release the fear and return to feeling calm and relaxed.

NOTE – For the technique to be effective, it is crucial that with your description of the situation during hypnosis you get the client to feel fear/anxiety.

Driving test nerves

Clients seeking therapy for driving test nerves are mostly young people. This will usually be conducted as a one-session therapy.

After inducing hypnosis use an IMR first to establish if there are any causes that may need to be looked at and dealt with.

You can use one, or a mix of the following techniques to help facilitate change and re-programming:
- Creating new behaviours.
- Visualisation.
- A driving test script.

Improving performance

Hypnosis can also be used to improve performance, whether it involves minimising nerves or simply perfecting and honing a skill. Clients might want to improve areas of performance such as:
- Sports performance
- Acting
- Music
- Dance
- Public speaking

When helping a client improve performance you must before hypnosis:

1. Establish what they want to achieve on the first session.

2. Make sure you establish the correct terminology to use when talking about their skill during hypnosis and make notes of this.

    e.g. Racquet rather than bat in tennis.

Improving performance generally involves more than one session.

Use IMR and regression if necessary. Useful scripts are available on improving performance.

If the client has had a previous bad experience, the following techniques can also be useful to facilitate change:
- Rewriting history
- Creating new parts
- Timeline

In this situation you may or may not need to use confidence therapy, depending on the client. Probably only around 20% of clients in this category require confidence therapy. If they are a confident sportsperson, for example, confidence will not be necessary.

Personal view: Deep-rooted problems

> I'd been working with special needs children but decided to train in hypnotherapy. Previously, my attitude to people with problems would be, 'Oh get on with it.' But after witnessing regression and issues around lack of confidence, for instance, now I realise that things can be so deep rooted and so far back some people are unable to just get on with it, so I definitely have a better understanding.

I thoroughly enjoyed that Lorraine allowed me to be me and not a hypnotherapy clone. As a result, we are hypnotherapists with our own personalities.

Steve Hayward

Summary

Whether dealing with a fear or improving performance it remains key that we focus on client-centred therapy, asking the right questions at the start to establish objectives and then remaining flexible to follow up with the appropriate change and reprogramming techniques.

Test yourself

Name the four levels of fear.

Explain the role of the ANS in fears/phobias.

Name a technique you could use to help a client with fear.

Fear of Being Alone

Mandy had such a fear of being on her own that she would stay in a relationship even if she was not happy. I followed the basic formula and the subconscious said it was necessary to look at the cause of the problem, which was aged 0 (when she was a baby).

I learnt a very valuable lesson with Mandy. As I teach that you never regress until you have installed a safe place, I dutifully counted from 1 to 7 suggesting she go to a pleasant place but when I asked where she was, she said, 'Nowhere.' We tried again with the same answer. Now this was in my early days and I helpfully (so I thought) suggested a nice beach. Bad idea! Mandy did not like the beach and unbeknown to both of us that was actually where her problem began.

After we did eventually come up with a safe place, we went back to the event that caused the problem. She was on Southsea Beach, a baby of five months. She said there was no one there, her mum had left her. At this point I was quite shocked but again I had jumped to the wrong conclusion. In fact her mum was taking a photo of her. Imagine the situation: a little baby on the beach felt abandoned, yet in an adult's mind she knew her mum was only taking a photo. Very often it is simply a misunderstanding.

It forever amazes me that so many hypnotherapists are terrified of regression. I did some Inner Child work and Gestalt to cut away the negative feelings. I delivered a very positive script and counted my client up. The after chat was fascinating. Mandy was 33 and she opened her eyes and said, 'I cannot believe it. I have been carrying that photo around with me all my life. It is at home in my top drawer. The funny thing is I look so miserable in the photo and I hate the clothes I am wearing. I am going home to throw it away.'

Dealing with causes can be paramount.

Toilet Anxiety

Toilet anxiety is quite a common problem and can be awful because it stops people going out for fear of not being able to get to a toilet. Jane worked for the NHS and her job was on the line as she was off sick a lot with anxiety. She would plan her route to work around toilets and tried to get there early to get a parking place close to the building. She would worry so much about it she would make herself ill.

During regression she went back to when she was seven and her mum was taking her to Brownies. When she was at the bus stop she wanted to go to the toilet but her mum said she had to wait as they would miss the bus. From there on she worried about what would happen if she wanted to go to the toilet and as an adult it affected her life.

We went on to build confidence and did lots of visualisation seeing herself confident during interviews at work as she did not want to cry. After the interviews a panel allocated her a parking space to make life easier.

I always remember Jane because hypnosis was so useful for her. Her job was fine and her employers congratulated themselves on allocating her a parking space because it had made her attendance so good. Jane said she sat there with her mouth open and wanted to say, 'Do you really think that a parking space solved my problem? I have been to a hypnotherapist!' She told me, 'I am really sorry Lorraine, but I didn't want to tell them and just let them think they'd solved my problem!'

Over the course of six or so appointments Jane's side effects were amazing. She felt confident, all of her aches and pains disappeared and she bounced into my office looking brilliant. She also went on to learn how to swim, something she had always wanted to do.

Fear of Lifts

Ann wanted to fly to America to visit friends. She was 63 had had a fear of lifts since getting stuck in one when she was 11. As people do, she had practised and practised her fear. Even though she told me her fear went back to getting stuck, I still followed the procedure and did IMR to find out if we needed to look at causes or not. I proceeded with the NLP fast phobia rewind technique, followed by positive suggestion. When I work with fears and phobias I like to make the next appointment after my client has had a chance to test if there have been any changes. It is very rare for a client to realise how serious their fear is and how much of their life it affects.

Ann was going to London on a coach trip and was also frightened of tunnels. The Hindhead Tunnel had just been built on the A3 and it was more than a mile long. A wonderful friend drove through it first and counted up to 85, so Ann could shut her eyes and know how long it lasted. The next time she went to London I suggested she keep her eyes open, to find out how she felt.

She came back so happy and told me she had been through the tunnel not only with her eyes open but with a smile on her face. Her husband Mike's face was a picture! It was the same with her fear of revolving doors. They arrived at their hotel and she felt really confident and just walked through. Apparently at this point she was laughing as Mike just stared with his mouth open. He could not believe what she had done. She said, 'So I did it again!'

We then went on to deal with causes. We did have to go back to the time when she was stuck in the lift and Ann got very upset. We did Inner Child then I taught her self-hypnosis to give her control so that if she did feel a panic attack she could do something about it. She was very confident lady and I felt she really needed to find out if she had her fear under control. She said her friends were coming over from America and she wanted to see if she could go in the lift all the way to the top of the Spinnaker Tower in Portsmouth.

I had the most wonderful phone call from her – she was so excited. I could hear her husband and her friends in the background and she had not only been up in the lift, she had also been down in the hull of HMS victory. She said, 'If you have anybody who doesn't believe in hypnosis, give them my phone number.' She was so pleased.

Chapter Thirteen

Habits and Addictions

More on Behaviours

This chapter takes us through habits and addictions:
- What they are? – Definitions.
- The psychology behind them and how they are formed.
- How we deal with them.

What is a habit? An action or pattern of behaviour that is repeated so often that it becomes typical of somebody, although he or she may be unaware of it.

What is an addiction? A state of physiological or psychological dependence to a substance or behaviour, slavery to a habit or vice.

Learned behaviour
Many psychological experiments have been conducted over the years to help us understand learned behaviours; as a hypnotherapist it is useful to have some knowledge of this background to have an insight into how habits and addictions are developed.

Researchers concluded that there are three main methods used in learning skills and these come under the general headings of Classical

Conditioning, Operant Conditioning and Cognitive Conditioning. We will also look at Learned Helplessness.

Classical Conditioning – Pavlov
Pavlov's experiment with dogs is one of the most famous.
- Pavlov's experiment was based on the premise that dogs salivate when presented with food.
- Each time he gave the dogs food he rang a bell.
- After a number of repetitions he did something different; he rang the bell but presented no food.
- He found that just the sound of the bell alone caused the dogs to salivate.
- The dogs had learned to respond to a stimulus, the bell.
- This type of learning is called Classical Conditioning.

Operant Conditioning – Skinner
Skinner used a device to train animals in a different way. The Skinner Box was used to deliver food to a pigeon based on it exhibiting the right behaviour.
- He found that if a pigeon was presented with food each time it pecked a red button it would learn to associate the red button with food and would peck the button whenever he wanted to eat.
- The box could be set to deliver food in different ways, either as above, at specific time intervals or randomly.
- A pigeon left overnight with the box set to deliver food at random intervals was found the next morning performing all kinds of movements in an effort to get food.
- He had learned incorrect associations with the delivery of food.
- It has been suggested that this is how superstitions develop.

Cognitive Conditioning
This is where previously learned skills can be used to make the learning of a new skill easier.

- A monkey is given a stick and learns to use it to reach a banana just out of his grasp.
- He then learns to use the stick to reach a longer stick so he can use it reach a banana even further away.
- The principles of the first task were used to help him learn a new skill.

Learned Helplessness

- A dog is placed in a Skinner Box where a few seconds after a bell is rung half of the floor becomes electrified. The dog learns to move quickly to the safe portion of the floor.
- Then the box is changed and as the bell rings the complete floor is electrified. There is no escape so the dog cowers in the corner.
- The box is changed to the original setting where only half the floor is electrified, yet the dog still cowers in the corner. He has learned to accept his fate: this is called learned helplessness.
- This has been associated with people in concentration camps. Many people with problems reach this state and so do not even seek help for their condition.

What has this got to do with hypnotherapy?
Repetition and reinforcement

The first three experiments demonstrate how we learn through repetition; each additional exposure to the event reinforces the learning and consolidates the skill. We develop habits through repetition, by practising a 'skill'.

Subconscious learning

When we learn something consciously we concentrate and purposefully focus our attention on achieving it.

Subconscious learning takes place in a different way. The subconscious is constantly monitoring our environment, processing lots of information and noticing things that we consciously ignore. So, many of the habits we learn are not consciously learned at all, they simply appear, such as anxiety and phobias.

Purposes of learning – conscious purposes
When we learn consciously we do so because we have a goal we view as desirable or beneficial.

Purposes of learning – subconscious purposes
The key goal of the subconscious is to defend itself and one of the main reasons for the subconscious to learn a skill is to relieve pressure caused by stress in the environment, real or perceived. This pressure can be relieved via one of two channels open to the subconscious, the physical body or psychological status. The problem arises when the subconscious believes it has dealt with the issue, but the conscious part of us does not like the outcome. This is the origin of the problem that brings a client for hypnotherapy.

Personal view: A journey of discovery
Lorraine quickly builds rapport and is one of the few people I can easily open up to. Her knowledge of the subject she teaches is excellent and her sense of humour makes even the dry topics interesting. Lorraine's informal, relaxed approach provides more than just a hypnotherapy course – it was a journey to discover even more about myself as an individual.

Jo Fellows, Kallisti Hypnotherapy

Tips for treating habits
Is the cause relevant?
When treating habits the original cause of the habit may not always be relevant.

Example: a person may have started smoking to look 'grown up' in front of friends – this original cause is unlikely to be relevant in the adult.

IMR can be used to establish whether we need to look at the cause or not. There may be other events we need to look at too. We need to ask the relevant questions with IMR to establish this.

Quitting a habit can leave a vacuum

When hypnotherapy is used to put an end to a habit we need to be aware that stopping a lifelong practice can leave a vacuum. This is why creating new behaviours and confidence therapy can be so important in helping to diminish this effect, by reprogramming with positive behaviours and approaches.

Addictions
Physiological dependency

When more and more of a drug is consumed the user needs more to achieve the same initial effect. When they stop taking the drug, the withdrawal symptoms can be described as side effects. Tolerance and withdrawal are linked to needs developed through subconscious learning.

Psychological dependency

This also develops through subconscious learning. A person can be dependent on a drug even though no physical need develops.

Example: a person may be dependent on a drug to relieve anxiety – alcohol or marijuana.

Psychological dependency can though move on to physiological dependency as more and more is consumed.

Treatment of addictions

There is a clear link between habits and addictions: both are learned responses. With addiction it is clear body chemistry is involved, however since the subconscious controls our body chemistry we can do something about it:
- Find the cause and its relevance.

- Use confidence therapy for reprogramming.
- Ensure your client cuts down on the drug gradually.
- A drug is like a crutch for a broken leg, you cannot take it away until the leg has mended.

Test yourself

Quitting a habit can leave a vacuum, what do we do in our therapy to prevent this?

If a client is taking any prescribed drugs for their problem, what is our stance?

Learned Behaviour – My Mum

I would like to touch again here on another issue of learned skills that we have already covered – learned behaviour. I will do so with a personal anecdote that I think offers us some valuable insights.

My mum was so lovely that although she did not understand my interest in hypnotherapy, she would humour me and let me practise on her. I remember one time in particular that she came to my therapy room and she sat in the chair and said, 'You have always been weird but I love you anyway.' I will always remember that as it made me smile.

My mum was very hard going as a 'client.' We worked with weight and whenever I tried to regress her she always said she did not know where she was. With experience, however, I used to manage to work with her and it turned out that all her life she felt unloved and unwanted with her family and friends. As I grew up with my mum I had an insight to her life, and the fact is that without consciously being aware of it my mum created scenarios that she wasn't wanted.

For example, she was a single parent mum, she shouted all the time and she was an aggressive parent. As children we learned we had to shout to be heard. As far as her brothers and sister were concerned, we were unruly children and we were not welcomed in their homes. Hence my mum produced her belief that she was not wanted. She just did not know how to be happy in her life, although I love her a great deal and she was the best mum she could have possibly been. She died young, at the age of 64. She was the life and soul of the party and her funeral was absolutely packed: they were standing outside. How's that for someone who believed she wasn't wanted? I remember saying, 'Look mum, how popular you are!'

Well, in therapy I used a lot of Inner Child and got my mum to love herself. It is so important to love yourself, even though it does sound corny. She did lose three stone before she died but would never admit that it was the hypnotherapy. My mum used to have a really shrill voice that could go right through you, and she lost that sound as well. There were other changes too. I was helping my business partner Steph to organise an art exhibition in our coffee shop in remembrance of her late daughter Rachel. I got so involved with the exhibition that I forgot to invite my mum until the Friday and the exhibition was on the Sunday. I quickly phoned her at work and said, 'I am really sorry but I forgot to tell you we are having an art exhibition for Rachel on Sunday, would you like to come?' To my pleasant surprise she said Yes. Before the hypnosis, she would have said. 'I don't know. I will see if I am doing anything.'

This is another example of how our subconscious does not analyse. It just produces a behaviour and repeats it. As far as it is concerned, the problem has been dealt with even if we are not consciously happy with it. My mum certainly wasn't, but she did not unlock the answer until her 'weird' daughter used hypnosis.

Chapter Fourteen

Working with Children

Working with children can be a joy and immensely rewarding, but needs to be approached very carefully. In this chapter we will:
- Clarify the law regarding the treatment of children.
- Describe the method for treating children.

Hypnosis and children – the law
First of all, it is important to state that it is not advisable to work with children under the age of seven as their concentration is not well enough developed for them to maintain focus long enough to respond to hypnotherapy.

Between the ages of seven and 14 an adult must be present during therapy. From the age of 14 the law states that a child can choose to be treated with or without the presence of a parent or adult.

Is treatment of the child appropriate?
Before beginning any treatment with a child you should establish if there is a problem to be treated in the first place.
- Often concerned parents may perceive problems that are really just part of normal behaviour.
- Or in fact the problem may be more related to the adult than the child; perhaps their behaviour is contributing to the problem.

Working with children – the method

1. *Before hypnosis* – The parent will usually begin by describing the child's problem. Once this has been established, focus on communicating directly with the child to build rapport.

2. A traditional induction cannot be used with children. Instead you need to create stories they can relate to and imagine so you grasp and maintain their attention. You need to chat to the child beforehand to find out what interests them, then build a story and the therapy around this.

3. Examples: walking a dog, horse-riding, going to the beach.

4. Dispel any fears by telling the child you are going to have some fun. You can relate the story telling and the use of their imagination to magic; children generally love the idea of magic.

5. *Inducing the trance* – Children have an amazing imagination, they love creative play, so as you begin to tell the story, ask them to close their eyes and say you are going to tell them a story. Say, 'Just picture it as I talk', refer to the magic of imagining so well that it seems real. Create an image that tires them out, like running: they become so exhausted they just flop down to take a rest, then they close their eyes and begin to dream.

6. *Assurance procedure* – You can use helium balloons on string, describing the balloons lifting their arm in the air and then when you cut the string, the arm just falls back to the chair.

7. ***Reprogramming*** – Continue with a story to facilitate their treatment. You can use IMR as usual, but often regression is not necessary because they are so young. You can just install a new programme, asking them to throw away the old one.

Conclusion

Working with children involves quite a different, specialised technique. If this is an area you would like to focus on, there are numerous courses available to help develop your skills further.

> **Test yourself**
>
> By law, at what age can a child choose to be treated without the presence of an adult?

Chapter Fifteen

Neurobiology

Neurobiology and hypnosis

Although a lot of the information in this chapter is very factual, I love it because it helps us understand what is actually happening in the brain. Sometimes when you are talking to clients under hypnosis it is reassuring to know that the way we think really does matter. I used to feel, 'Who am I? Does this really work? All I am doing is talking! How can this help someone?'

Well, in this chapter we are going to take a look at neurobiology to develop our understanding of how hypnosis works, and we will discover how 'thought' actually changes the chemistry in the brain.

This evidence is crucial to us as hypnotherapists as, studies of the brain and nervous system and how they function provide factual evidence that back up the power of hypnotherapy. They substantiate theories about how hypnosis creates genuine changes and benefits for our clients – and they provide a resounding answer to those who falsely claim hypnosis is no more than a confidence trick.

As hypnotherapists we therefore have a *proven scientific base* to reiterate the good we can *see* we are doing!

How hypnosis works
- Structure of the nervous system
- Neuroplasticity
- The brain and memory
- Explanation of the effects of hypnosis on brain function

Structure of the nervous system

The nervous system can be split into two main parts:
1. The brain and central nervous system.

2. The peripheral nervous system.

Neurons

The brain, along with the rest of the nervous system, is made up of neurons. Neurons are a very specialist type of cell. They only exist to activate each other or other cells within the brain or body.

Here's a diagram of a neuron. Nerve impulses are picked up from a source then passed along between neurons to carry out a job – making a muscle contract, for example.

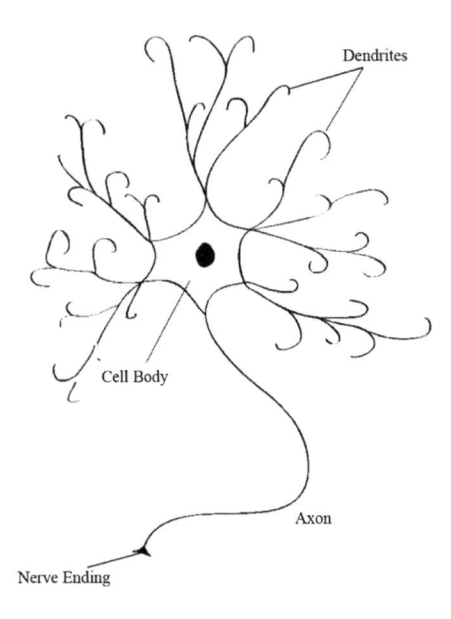

The Neuron

Dendrites are branches attached to the cell body. They pick up nerve impulses from other neurons or sensors. The nerve impulses pass through the cell body and then along the length of the axon to the nerve ending, always travelling in the same direction. Impulses travel through chains of neurons connected through the nerve ending attached to the dendrites of the next neuron.

The terminal neuron may be attached to a muscle by a muscle end plate and this will then operate the contraction of the muscle.

The Axon

Axons are surrounded by a myelin sheath that insulates the slender nerve fibres and speeds up the transmission of nerve impulses.

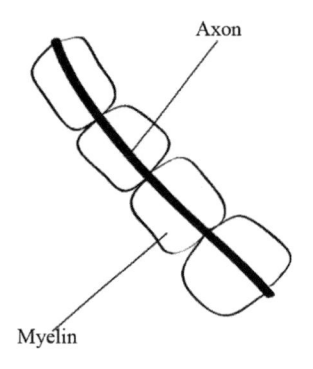

Nerve impulses are chemical reactions – these are neurotransmitters. The axon is rich in potassium and myelin is rich in sodium. During the transmission of an impulse, the two chemicals react. In fact, the nervous system uses many neurotransmitters and each chemical is used for a specific job.

There are drugs (for example Prozac) that imitate the action of these chemicals and force the brain to act in a particular way. However, as these chemicals are not the actual neurotransmitters, they can act on more than one site and cause other effects. They can also interact with other chemicals naturally occurring in the body and again cause side effects.

Let us just take a pause here and think about multiple sclerosis.

Multiple Sclerosis and hypnotherapy

Axons can be incredibly long – up to 3ft – which means that as cells, some neurons are real giants. To protect these slender fibres, and speed up the transmission of an impulse over such a long distance (if you have just touched something red hot, for example), axons are covered in a sheath of myelin that acts like the plastic cable around electrical wires.

It is the myelin sheath that is damaged in MS. Without its protection, the neuron cannot fire properly, leading to jerkiness and co-ordination trouble. Unlike other cells, science says that under normal circumstances neurons cannot regenerate, so MS is considered incurable.

With hypnotherapy, however, we can help MS patients with a lot of success. The reason is that subconscious mind is responsible (as we saw in Chapter Two) for maintaining and operating the physical body, and having built myelin when it first built the brain and nervous system, it still knows how to do it. By talking to the subconscious mind we can ask it to make more. Some patients appear to have made a permanent recovery after hypnotherapy, although legally we have to say that they are in remission rather than cured.

The brain and CNS

This picture shows a cross section of the brain.

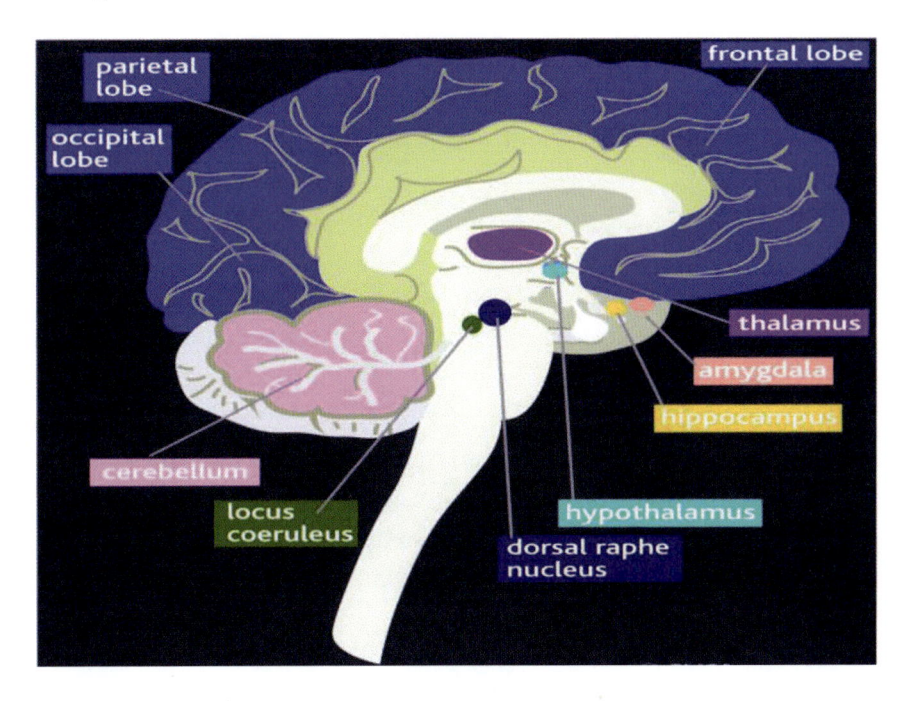

It is split into two halves known as hemispheres. The two hemispheres are divided into areas known as lobes. They are connected by a thick cable of axons that allows the two sides to talk to each other. Psychologists have done various studies of people who have had this link surgically severed, usually for epilepsy treatment. Known as 'split brain' studies, they show how even though the brain is in two halves, they exchange information between the two hemispheres to create a whole.

The lobes have been identified as having associations with different functions: for example, the occipital lobe has been linked to visual processing, and the temporal to language. Here's another fascinating example: a part of the brain called the ventromedial hypothalamus determines when we have had enough to eat, and it is possible under hypnosis to suggest that a client with weight problems will feel satisfied after eating less. This suggestion adjusts the levels set in the ventromedial hypothalamus so the client stops eating sooner.

The peripheral nervous system

The peripheral nervous system is split into two halves, the somatic system and the visceral system.

The somatic system controls the sensory and motor nervous systems. This is principally concerned with skin, muscles and joints.

The skin contains nerves and receptors for heat, pain, pressure, electrical activity, chemicals and body position. All these things tell us information about our environment. We all know what goose bumps feel like; this is either a response to receptors on the skin responding to cold air by erecting the hairs on our skin, or an emotional response that causes the same physical response due to a memory. Our mind records all these physical feelings as well as external elements of the environment all the time.

The visceral nervous system is also known as the Autonomic Nervous System or ANS. The role of the ANS is to control the various metabolic functions within the body. For example, heart rate and blood pressure, to keep the body comfortable. The ANS has two parts:
- The sympathetic nervous system, which prepares the body for emergency action (the 'fight or flight' response).
- The parasympathetic nervous system, which restores normality.

These should balance to maintain equilibrium within the body's metabolic functions, but if the sympathetic system is more powerful the person will be edgy, anxious and tense. If the parasympathetic system has the upper hand, the person may be depressed and lethargic. When the equilibrium is upset permanently, this manifests itself in physical and mental conditions such as stress or phobia. Hypnotherapy can treat these conditions and restore balance.

Neuroplasticity

'Neurons that fire together, wire together'

Canadian psychologist Donald Hebb

Neuroplasticity is the ability to adapt and reshape our brain and its pathways. It occurs inside us every day as we encounter new experiences. The brain is a very malleable organ. It can and does change its structure throughout our lives.

An example of neuroplasticity is sensory substitution. For example, if a person is born blind, often the visual parts of the brain will be taken over by another sense, such as hearing or touch.

This is the brain's way of re-allocating unused processing power to what we are actually experiencing. It would be wasteful to leave potential neural networks dormant simply because we weren't getting any input from that sense. Our brains have evolved over time to become more adaptive to these changes in our biology.

The brain and memory

A memory trace in the brain is known as an engram. Lots of research has been done over the years to try to locate where memories are made or stored in the brain.

It has been found that the area known as the hippocampus, along with the temporal lobe and other areas of the neo-cortex, are all used together to record everything that happens when a memory is being stored. This includes smells and sounds. We all know how a smell can take us right back to a place we remember, whether it is soggy school dinners or a flower-filled garden, and this is why. There is an actual physical storage of the information that the subconscious has recorded.

So when we regress clients and take them back into that moment, they can see, feel and experience the events, exactly as they did at the time. This is easy to understand when you realise that all of these things are actually recorded in the brain at the time.

Effects of hypnosis on the brain
Can we see what effect hypnosis has on the brain?

Our brainwaves and the patterns they make can be illustrated by EEG (electroencephalogram) printouts. When we are wide awake we usually show beta waves. We move through alpha waves until we pass through theta waves and on to delta waves when we reach deep asleep.

Under hypnosis, we exhibit alpha waves as we start to relax and become calm. During the induction these fade and are replaced with theta and delta waves. This continues under the deepening process. During therapy, the waves change, becoming mostly delta and some theta waves. As we awaken alpha waves increase whilst delta and theta fade, after which beta waves return to previous levels as we awaken.

What does this mean? Brainwave information is not a definitive indicator of how the mind is operating, but this pattern does fit the hypothesis that the conscious mind backs off during hypnosis and the subconscious mind takes a more active role.

What is more, under hypnosis it has been shown that the brains of subjects show less activity in the left hemisphere, the logical reasoning centre of the brain. In contrast, there is an increase in the activity levels in the right hemisphere, the centre for imagination and creativity.

While this is not conclusive evidence, it does support the idea that hypnotism opens up the subconscious mind. Recent brain studies of people who are susceptible to suggestion show that when they act on the suggestions their brains show profound changes in how they process information. The suggestions literally change what people see, hear, feel and believe to be true.

When we work with our clients to create new behaviours or change memories, we are actually having a physical effect on the brain structure. We are in effect enabling our client to change their neuron pathways and create new behaviours. This is reinforced by the recordings we give out, which take our clients again and again down this new pathway.

Eventually, the old behaviours from the old pathway will fade. As the pathway falls out of use, there is the chance of the brain reusing this area for another function and the old pathway ceases to exist. This is why reinforcement is so important. Our client needs to keep using the new pathway for it to become embedded and become the 'normal/usual' behaviour.

The fact is, what we think does really matter, and thought changes the chemistry in the brain. Roger Sleet has written about the implications of this in his excellent book, *'A Guide to Professional Hypnotherapy'* and I would like to quote an excerpt of it here.

Hypnotherapists – beware

"Hypnotherapy deals with reality. The therapist should realise that although the therapy is aimed at the mind, it alters the chemistry of the nervous system. When the mind performs an action, no matter how trivial, the first tangible evidence we have that anything has happened is that a chemical is realised in the brain.

One thought will cause a set of neurons to release their neurotransmitters. Hearing one spoken word will also activate neurons. In other words, hypnotherapy is not just a 'psychological' therapy: it is also a physical therapy. Suggestions produce physical changes.

To take this principle to its extreme, we could also follow other lines of logic. Spoken words will produce activity in the auditory areas of the temporal lobes. This will be fed back up to the mind for processing, also producing activity in the association areas. The way in which this information is processed in the mind will determine what will result as the chemical status of the nervous system, which in turn will have its effect on the physical body.

If a person is continuously exposed to negative input to the extent that they begin to think habitually in a depressing way, then this will cause certain neurons to fire. Neurotransmitters are specific to the job the neurons have to do. Therefore a very specific chemical will be found in abundance in the brain.

On the other hand, if the input is positive, and the person is habitually cheerful, a completely different set of chemicals are involved. The spoken word is therefore a powerful thing. It alters the chemistry of the brain and produces positive or negative effects.

It is vital that therapists of any kind be aware of this. Every word spoken in the presence of a client, whether hypnosis is involved or not, should be very positive in nature.

If negativity is not removed, it could actually cause more damage. On the other hand, positive conversation actually assists the healing processes."

Taken from A Guide to Professional Hypnotherapy, by Roger Sleet

The relaxed brain and the active brain

Take a look at the four pictures here.

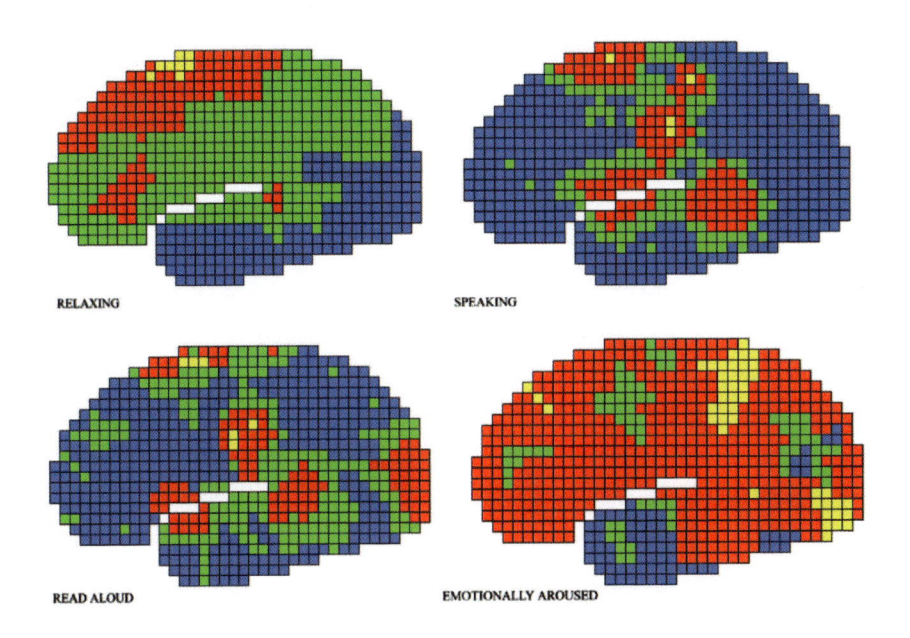

RELAXING

SPEAKING

READ ALOUD

EMOTIONALLY AROUSED

They illustrate how active different parts of the brain are, according to this colour code:
- Blue – very little activity
- Green – average activity
- Red – a lot of activity
- Yellow – intense activity.

The pictures were taken using a scanner and measuring activity by the amount of blood supply being sent to different parts of the brain. Let us just compare the relaxed brain with the emotionally active brain.

Relaxed brain Even though this person is relaxing with their eyes closed, their hearing, smell and some sensory areas are all still active and show up with red patches, while the association areas are also buzzing as he or she thinks their own thoughts. The predominant colour, however, is green.

Emotionally aroused brain Here there is a lot of intense activity, shown by reds and yellows as the mind whirrs. This person looks like they have a problem weighing down on them.

The important point is that the activated areas are very similar between the two pictures, which is significant for hypnotherapists. It is just a case of changing the colours. If we could put the emotional person under hypnosis, they would change from red to green, where they would be far more receptive to suggestion.

What this indicates is that there is a physical side to any psychological problem, something that has big implications for treatment.

Drugs

Whereas the medical profession prefers to treat psychological problems with psychoactive drugs, the approach of hypnotherapy is completely different.

These drugs travel in the bloodstream, and blood supply in the brain varies according to how much activity is taking place at different times. This means that there is no telling exactly where the drug will go, which neurons it will activate and what reaction it will produce in the body, hence the problem of side effects.

For those who would like a more technical description of this phenomenon, I have included here a diagram likening the effects to a lock and key as molecules of psychoactive drugs known as 'blockers' and 'depressants' hunt down receptor sites that will stop neurons firing. They aim to dampen down the nervous system to reduce hyperactivity and anxiety. Drugs known as 'stimulants', on the other hand, gets neurons sparking in patients suffering from apathy and depression.

The Lock and Key Mechanism

Just as a key has to be the right shape to fit a lock, a molecule has to be the right shape to fit the receptor in order for it to work.

A typical neurotransmitter has a receptor, represented in the diagram on the left. When a molecule of exactly the right shape and size attaches to the receptor, as shown by the diagram on the right, the receptor will fire. Other neurotransmitters have different-shaped receptors that attach to different-shaped molecules. This ensures that only the correct receptors fire to pass specific messages along.

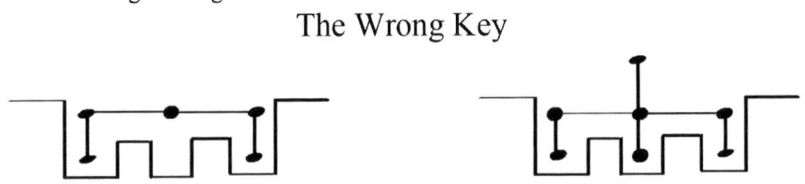

The Wrong Key

If a molecule of the wrong shape attaches to a receptor, as shown in the diagram on the left, then the neuron cannot fire. It also prevents the correct molecules from attaching to the receptor site. This is what happens with drugs known as depressants or blockers, which are designed to prevent neurons from firing. They are used to suppress hyperactivity.

If a drug has a molecule that fits a receptor, even though it is the wrong shape, as shown in the diagram on the right, the neuron will fire. This is how stimulants work. These are chemicals that mimic natural neurotransmitters and fire neurons when there is a shortage of the appropriate molecules.

The Wrong Lock

A receptor was discovered with an unusual shape that did not fit any of the standard neurotransmitters. It was found to fit certain opiate drugs. Yet surely man was not designed to be an opium addict! With further research it was discovered that these receptors were the right shape to fit endorphins, a chemical found naturally in the body.

Hypnotherapy is different. It does not just tackle symptoms. Unlike with drugs or needles (in acupuncture), it uses the spoken word to establish and deal with causes, and helps to remove symptoms at source. As Roger Sleet writes:

" Since the spoken word produces changes in the brain, this tool can be used to make the brain produce specific chemicals at specific sites...

This research gives the hypnotherapist confidence that this form of therapy is not just a flight of fancy, or a confidence trick. This is reality. The therapy influences the mind. This produces chemical changes in the body. Hypnotherapy can be used to bring about changes anywhere in this chain of command, making it very valuable therapy indeed."

Test yourself

Name the two halves of the ANS.

What is the normal functioning role of the ANS?

Chapter Sixteen

Psychophysiological Disorders

Medical Classifications

You will have seen by now that hypnosis can help with a wide variety of conditions. You may be wondering why and how, so this chapter investigates how illness is created in the first place.

Causes of illness
There are only three ways to be unwell:
1. A collision with the environment e.g. an accident leading to a cut finger or broken leg.

2. The body is invaded by a virus or bacteria.

3. The mind creates it.

If the illness/condition is not the result of a collision with the environment or a virus, then it must have been created by the mind. If this is the case, the condition has been created by the subconscious.

What can hypnotherapy change?
- Hypnotherapy can cure anything in category 3
- Hypnotherapy can help with category 1, by speeding up the body's healing process.
- A virus will need to run its own course, although its effects can sometimes be minimised by hypnotherapy.

Definition: *A psychophysiological illness is 'a physical illness that has psychological causes.'*

> **Fascinating fact:** Eight million people live with chronic pain. But with a combination of drugs, surgery, physio and psychological treatment, it can be beaten.
>
> *Source: Daily Mail*

It is important to note that the physical symptom is real and not imagined.
e.g. An ulcer is a physical condition, yet its cause is psychological.

Note – Do not confuse this with conversion or hysterical reactions. In this case the physical aspect is imaginary (and so psychological).
e.g. hysterical blindness or paralysis.

When you are working with clients, you will need to feel comfortable with the presenting problem. If you feel unsure, do not work with them. Check they have been seen by a medical professional, as sometimes a headache can be the mind telling them they have a brain tumour. Most people, however, have usually been down a few roads before trying hypnosis. My advice is to be sure.

I have worked with depression and my clients have been on medication at the time of the therapy. I never advise any of them to come off their medication without the help of their doctor. One client, Faye, was working with me with depression and she had been on antidepressants for a couple of years. After a couple of sessions with me she went to her doctor and she seemed so much happier that he asked her what we she was on. She explained she was seeing me. He said: 'Well, it certainly seems to be helping you. Let's start reducing your dose.' By the end of our therapy, Faye was totally drug free and enjoying her life.

I would also advise that you do not work with clients presenting schizophrenia or psychopathic personality.

How can the mind create an illness?
If we think back to the functions of the subconscious mind, we have our answer. These functions are:
- The maintenance and the operation of the physical body.
- The development of habits and skills.
- The storage and retrieval of memories.

All of these interact.
The mind is the controller sending messages to the brain and nervous system that then create physical changes in the body.

Psychological problem – a disturbance in the mind, the effects of which can be seen in the brain.

Psychophysiological problem – where a physical condition has been created by the subconscious. It is also a disturbance of the mind but its effects can be seen in both the brain and the body. This is also known as a psychosomatic illness.

The mechanics of the mind's influence
Now let us take a look at some specific examples of how the mind influences the body via the brain and nervous system.

Muscle control, blood flow and pressure

Tension, often caused by stress, is a common factor in blood pressure problems. Tension makes the muscles contract, as the neurons that end in the muscles are activated; they then squeeze the blood vessels, increasing blood pressure. This often leads to headaches, migraines and other high blood pressure conditions. As tension causes the involuntary contraction of muscles this can also lead to pain in the neck and shoulders or knotted up sensations in the stomach.

Imbalance of the autonomic nervous system

The perception of stress or danger leads to the activation of the sympathetic division of the ANS, creating the fight or flight response, which causes chemical and physical changes in the body. This is a necessary function designed for short-term gain but if this abnormal state continued it could lead to problems so the parasympathetic system therefore acts to calm things down and restore normality, as we saw in Chapter Fifteen.

A psychological state of wariness upsets the balance of this system; it keeps the sympathetic system slightly activated, thereby releasing chemicals that are not really needed. These chemicals as they circulate around the body can have a negative effect because they are acidic or alkaline in nature. They attack body tissue and can be the cause of an ulcer. Other effects of an imbalance of the ANS can be high blood pressure, shortage of breath and palpitations.

Eating behaviour

Thought is chemical: being happy involves the creation of one kind of chemical, being depressed or unhappy involves the creation of another. Raw materials in the form of food are required to create these chemicals and so can create fancies, the body's way of telling you what you need. Being on a diet can cause frustration when you cannot quell these needs; the lack of certain necessary raw materials can then lead to other physical conditions.

Cell manufacture and regeneration
Our subconscious mind controls the cells of our body, making sure they are replaced at regular intervals (except neurons). When the subconscious gets this wrong mutated cells are produced, causing illness such as cancer.

Healing
As the subconscious mind controls the body's healing mechanisms, a change in the psychological state can cause the healing mechanisms to speed up or slow down, having an impact on how much and how well healing happens.

Energy field
As we know, the subconscious mind controls our energy field, the pathway to the body that does not involve the brain and nervous system. This field can be manipulated and can, for example, bring about changes in body shape when dealing with weight problems.

In summary, we can see that the mind can create a wide range of physical conditions simply by using the mechanisms at its disposal. So the reverse is also true, and the subconscious mind can heal these conditions – this is where hypnotherapy can help.

Warning
Some psychophysiological conditions are life threatening, such as cancer or a tumour. They may be the result of a subconscious decision to end the person's life. For obvious reasons new therapists should not attempt to deal with these cases.

Treating psychophysiological disorders
Treatment involves using the usual basic formula detailed in Chapter Eight.

Psychological problem – dealt with by establishing the cause using IMR and regression if necessary.

Physical symptoms – healing can be helped by visualisation, NLP techniques and healing scripts. (Technical anatomical knowledge is not necessary as the subconscious mind has all the knowledge and tools it needs.) Healing takes time, so CDs will help back up the process, along with remembering the fourth rule of suggestion: 'Be patient'.

> **Fascinating fact:** NHS guidelines allow doctors to refer patients with irritable bowel syndrome for hypnotherapy or other psychological therapies to ease the symptoms if medication is unsuccessful and the problem persists.
> *Source: NHS*

Test yourself

Name the three ways to be unwell.

What is the definition of a psychophysiological illness?

Healing the Hairdresser

I am really family orientated and whenever my daughter Rachel's friends are round, I just cannot help myself.

Hayleigh used to get a sty every month, but since I treated her she has not produced a single one in three years. Which is just as well, as she is about to get married and would definitely have had a sty on her big day.

I helped Hayleigh one evening, when I came home at 9pm to find all my daughter's friends having a girlie night in the lounge. Knowing I am a hypnotherapist, Hayleigh asked if I could do anything with her sty. She looked at me and she had the most awful sty on her eye. It was huge and she was hiding it behind her sweeping fringe. The doctors had said they could not help.

I took Hayleigh upstairs to my therapy room. I had known her since she was a teenager so I already had a good rapport with her. We sat and had a pre-chat. She is a very ambitious young girl, a mobile hairdresser and beauty therapist who works long hours, which is stressful. She wanted the sty gone by Monday as she was going up to London with friends. I said I would ask if the sty could be gone by Monday.

I took Hayleigh into hypnosis and asked her to choose a finger and then I got an IMR response. I asked subconscious mind is there was anything we needed to look at to help her let go of the sty. The answer was Yes.

We went back to when she was ten and her grandmother had died. I did Inner Child and gestalt. I said, 'Subconscious, you know how to make this sty? You know how to unmake it?' I asked if it could unmake it by Monday. 'Yes.' I asked it to make all the adjustments necessary and let me know when it was ready.

I waited, delivered some very positive suggestions and counted Hayleigh up from hypnosis. We went and joined the girls downstairs.

On Wednesday night Hayleigh came round to find me. She said: 'I forgot all about the hypnosis and I got into bed on Sunday night. Oh, you would never believe it! My sty popped and there wasn't one but two. It was disgusting. All this green stuff came out. It was horrible. I woke up on Monday morning and it was gone. Isn't that amazing?'

No Point Being Ill

The way we all learn is from our parents, teachers, friends and family. We learn from watching and hearing things said to us, and this is all stored in our subconscious mind, where we learn our behaviours.

My daughter Rachel was chatting to one of her friends and as I walked past her bedroom door I heard her say, 'There is no point in being ill, my mum never takes any notice of you!' Which is true, and it did make me smile. When Rachel and her brother were young and they had colds and stomach upsets, I would say to them, 'That's alright. You will feel better at school.' The truth is, I do think you will feel better if you get up and go rather than lying around feeling sorry for yourself. Both of my children had a high attendance record at school – some years it would be 100% and now they are very rarely ill.

My friend Jane had three children and one or other of them was always off school. I told her I had never known such ill children. We worked together for a number of years and I got to know the family quite well. One of them would either have an earache, stomach ache, cough or cold. I would watch Jane fuss over them – she gave them a lot of attention. One day I was chatting to her daughter and asked about her stomach aches and she said she had double English that day!

Without consciously realising it she was making herself ill, not really the way she wanted attention.

MEDICAL CLASSIFICATIONS

In this section I would like to outline what is generally meant by terms such as stress and frustration, describe some defence mechanisms that come into play when we are in a stressful situation, and list common classifications of abnormal behaviour (although what actually defines normal/abnormal behaviour is a matter of debate among medical professionals and therapists, as I am sure you can imagine.)

Stress

Every single one of us has to deal with stress; it is a part of life, a normal function, and without it we become bored or listless. But each of us develops different ways of responding to that stress and how we deal with it has an impact on the quality of our life and our state of health. Causes of stress include:

Frustration

We all encounter obstacles in life:

- Obstacles from the physical environment (traffic jams)
- Obstacles from the social environment (disagreements)
- Obstacles caused by personal limitations (inadequate self control, physical handicap)

When these obstacles block or delay our progress towards a goal, we become frustrated.

Conflict

Frustration occurs when two motives conflict. Most conflicts involve goals that are both desirable and undesirable:
   e.g. chocolate is delicious but fattening.
   e.g. sexual desires versus moral standards.

Reactions to frustration
Aggression
Direct aggression is aimed at the object or person causing the frustration. This aggression can be physical or more often verbal. Aggression can be a learned way of solving a problem.

Displaced aggression occurs when a person cannot attack the object of frustration, perhaps because they were brought up not to hit people, or because the cause is not a concrete thing. They still need to attack something so they direct their aggression at a scapegoat.
- **Regression** – the individual returns to an immature behaviour that has been successful in the past when attempts to solve a problem fail. e.g. sulking
- **Apathy** – refer to 'learned helplessness' in Chapter Thirteen.
  Anxiety – many words can be used in the place of anxiety e.g. worry, dread, apprehension, fear.

Established disciplines consider anxiety to be the root of all psychological problems.

Defence mechanisms
The purpose of a defence mechanism is to change the way a person thinks about an anxiety-provoking situation. It distorts reality and often involves self-deception.

1. Denial
If we do not wish to face the problem or situation we may deny that it exists.

2. Repression
This is where we shut painful memories out from our consciousness.

3. Rationalisation
This is where we justify our behaviour making it conform to socially desirable motives.
e.g. I bought the new car because the old one would have had problems soon.

4. Projection
We protect ourselves by comparing ourselves to others.
e.g. At least my dyed hair looks more natural than hers.

5. Reaction formation
This is where you pretend to have an opposite view.
e.g. If you do not like someone you may actually be overly nice to them to try to conceal your true thoughts.

6. Intellectualisation
If a situation could be potentially emotionally distressing, intellectualisation is used to detach from it.
e.g. A doctor considering a patient as a number or case.
e.g. Politicians considering soldiers as numbers.

7. Displacement
If a motive cannot be directly satisfied then displacement involves satisfying it via any alternative method.
e.g. Taking up a sport to work out aggression rather than lashing out.

Abnormal behaviour
As I mentioned at the start of this section, some stress is necessary for normal functioning, however when it becomes too intense or prolonged then it can have a detrimental impact psychologically or physiologically. The three main

classes of psychological illness, as defined by the medical profession, are:

1. Neuroses
2. Psychoses
3. Personality disorders

Classifying abnormal behaviour

1. Neuroses
Troublesome enough to require expert help, and occasionally hospitalisation is necessary, but they do not involve personality disintegration or loss of contact with reality. Neurotics can usually get along in society, even though they do not function at full capacity. The primary symptom is anxiety.
- **Anxiety reactions**
- **Obsessive-compulsive reactions**
- **Phobias**
- **Conversion reactions**
- **Neurotic depression**

2. Psychoses
Characterised by an impairment in mental functioning that seriously interferes with the person's ability to meet the demands of life. There is gross distortion of reality, so that the person cannot distinguish between fantasy and reality. These distortions may take the form of delusions or hallucinations. A psychotic may also show profound changes of mood as well as defects in language and memory.

There are two general categories of psychoses, organic and functional:

Organic psychoses result from damage to the nervous system. Head injuries, brain tumours, hardening of the arteries, and lead poisoning are some of the conditions that can produce psychotic symptoms.

Functional psychoses are disorders that are presumed to be primarily psychological in origin, although genetic and biological factors may well play a part.
- **Manic states**
- **Depressive states**
- **Manic depression** (now called 'bipolar affective disorder')
- **Schizophrenia**

3. Personality disorders
These are a group of behaviours that are maladaptive more from society's viewpoint than in terms of the person's own discomfort or unhappiness. Extreme dependency, antisocial or sexually deviant behaviour, alcoholism and drug dependency are included here. There is no gross distortion of reality or intellectual impairment.
- **Psychopathic personality**
- **Alcoholism and drug dependence**

Methods of treatment
Drugs
There are a number of psychoactive drugs used in the treatment of psychological conditions e.g. Valium, Activan, Librium. It is useful to have a drug directory (MIMS) to gain a basic understanding of any drugs your client may be taking.

Counselling and group therapy
This can include psychiatrists, mental nurses or social workers for example, working with individuals or in groups.

Electroconvulsive therapy (ECT)
ECT has also been used in the treatment of these conditions and has been surrounded by controversy.

Chapter Seventeen

Setting Up in Business

You have slaved over your books and notes, practised and practised, made mistakes and learned from them, honed your techniques and grown in confidence. Now you are ready to make a career of the fascinating and fulfilling profession that is hypnotherapy. Yes, you are on your way!

Few hypnotherapy manuals cover the practical information you need to actually start your own business, but to me it is vital to get this right. It will give you a valuable head start. So in this chapter I have included everything you need to know to set yourself up in business as a hypnotherapist:
- Qualifications
- Professional support
- Insurance
- Setting up your office/therapy room
- Professional conduct and NOS Standards
- Accounts and taxation requirements
- Marketing

Qualifications and Professional Support
Students who have passed my Hampshire School of Hypnotherapy training course are entitled to add the following after their name

on any literature: Dip HSH. Other recognised courses should have similar rules.

General Hypnotherapy Register (GHR)

The **GHR** is currently the largest professional registering organisation for practising hypnotherapists in the UK. Apart from the professional credibility that registration bestows, they also provide a wide range of regularly updated membership benefits. They are additionally the administrators for the **General Hypnotherapy Standards Council (GHSC)**, which currently represents more than 180 separate professional bodies and training schools. The GHSC is responsible for overseeing the criteria for the ongoing registration of individual practitioners within the GHR and for the assessment and validation of hypnotherapy training courses that lead to that registration. The GHSC/GHR is a self-regulated governing body recognised both nationally and internationally.

Benefits

- Affiliation with the UK's largest professional association for practising hypnotherapists.
- The acquisition of a standardised, professional award, the General Qualification in Hypnotherapy Practice (GQHP) or if applicable, the Senior version (SQHP).
- A listing on their website and links to your own.
- Permission to use their logo on all marketing.
- A useful newsletter each month.
- Membership of the GHR is required if you wish to work with business organisations and their employees.
- William Broom, the head of the organisation, is very approachable and will provide advice on key professional matters (not general practice queries or where the answer is easily obtainable elsewhere).

For further details take a look at their website: www.general-hypnotherapy-register.com

Membership of the Hampshire School of Hypnotherapy (HSH)

Students who have trained with me are eligible for three years of support and help with any questions they may have. They are also eligible to join the HSH.

Benefits

- Access to the online forum, where you can obtain help/advice from other therapists.
- A 'rolling' listing on the main site, so visitors can find a therapist in their area.
- Affiliates to Twitter, Facebook and LinkedIn.
- Updates on current trends in hypnotherapy.
- Useful tools posted on the website.
- Quarterly meetings.
- Updates with opportunities for continual professional development and ad-hoc courses.

A small membership fee is payable.

Why join? HSH backs and supports former students as practising hypnotherapists, while the GHR provides credibility as a renowned professional governing body.

How can you describe your profession?

You can simply call yourself a hypnotherapist or you can use the term clinical hypnotherapist, as this simply means that you read scripts. You can, if you choose, use the term 'hypnotherapist using psychotherapy and NLP techniques.'

Insurance

Your only legal requirement as a hypnotherapist is to purchase insurance. I recommend you choose a company that provides legal cover as part of their package. A sample policy is provided in the Appendix.

Setting up your office/therapy room
For a welcome, practical therapy room you will need:
- Comfy chair – a recliner is ideal (do not use a bed).
- Blanket – for modesty (covering legs), warmth and comfort.
- Box of tissues – hypnotherapy and emotion go hand in hand.
- Toilet easily accessible.
- A quiet environment without any major noise.
- Recording equipment.
- Appointment book.
- A place to file client records.
- Informal layout to seating – two chairs at an angle makes people feel more comfortable (rather than directly opposite with a barrier in between).

I always advise that, if it is possible, you set up a room in your house, as this will keep costs down. You can be professional in your home. The advantage is that it is very private, and you can make people feel at home and in a very safe environment. Make sure your room is warm and clean. Later, when you are busy, you can look into acquiring business premises.

Professional conduct
Hypnotherapy is a professional occupation, so it is important to present a professional image to your clients at all times.
- Personal appearance smart, casual.
- Polite and courteous approach.
- Flexible and adaptable approach to people.
- Keep the therapy room clean.
- Avoid any strong perfume or other lingering fragrances like incense or oils. Sense of smell is heightened during hypnosis and the aromas may trigger unpleasant memories.
- Maintain and file client records confidentially. Do not write anything down you would not be happy for your client to read.

Client confidential records
- Each client must have their own record created and maintained. (A sample form is included in the Appendix).
- These records are confidential, to be seen only by you and your client. If a doctor requests a copy, you must obtain written permission from your client before passing on any information.

NOTE – Hypnotherapists do not need to seek permission from a client's doctor before providing treatment.

– Doctors cannot legally recommend that a patient see a hypnotherapist. However, it is acceptable for them to do so and occasionally some will let you put your leaflets in their surgery.

National Occupational Standards
As part of our professional conduct as specified by the GHSC, all therapists need to be aware of and abide by the National Occupational Standards:
- Complementary and Natural Healthcare Council NOS – Principles of Good Practice.
- CNH1: Explore and establish clients' needs for complementary and natural healthcare.
- CNH2: Develop and agree plans for complementary and natural healthcare with clients.
- CH-HI: Principles of Good Practice.
- CNH23: Provide Hypnotherapy to Clients.

To obtain a copy of the National Occupational Standards follow the link http://nos.ukces.org.uk/Pages/index.aspx and in the search enter Hypnotherapy. This will give you a copy of the standards laid out by the CNHC.

Accounts and taxation requirements

When you first set up in business as 'self employed' it will probably be most economical and easy enough to complete your own accounts. This is what you need to do:

1. Phone the tax office and ask for a tax reference number.

2. You can register for self assessment online. It will take just half an hour to fill out your tax return at the end of the year.

3. You need to record your sales and your expenses then at the end of the year deduct your expenses from your sales to establish your profit. Sample accounts are provided in the Appendix to give you an idea of what to do.

4. You can record your expenses and sales either in a book or on a simple Microsoft Excel spreadsheet. Keep all receipts as evidence of expenses in case they are requested at any time.

Marketing

I am sure by now you have some of your own ideas on how you will market your service. Here are some ideas and tips to get you started. These have worked well for me:

- A website is a must. (People are most likely to 'Google' for a hypnotherapist rather than look in a directory)
- Join networking clubs.
- Use social networking e.g. Twitter, Facebook.
- Blogging.
- Newspapers – you need to have a rolling plan so people see your name regularly. Try to get a free editorial to accompany your advert.
- Talks.
- Referrals.
- Testimonials – get into the habit of asking for them.
- Collect your clients' email addresses and keep in contact with them quarterly.

In my experience, leaflet drops tend to have a very low response rate, though if you hit the same area time and time again this may yield a better result.

Advertising Standards

Contrary to what many people believe, the Advertising Standards Authority actually has no legal authority if anyone complains about your adverts or website. If they receive a complaint you will receive a letter advising you of the complaint along with suggested changes to your literature. If you choose, you can simply make alterations as suggested.

To avoid any complaints the simple rule to remember is to avoid making any promises or guarantees. As an example:
DO NOT SAY – Hypnotherapy **will** cure …
DO SAY – Hypnotherapy can **help** with …

For advice on getting your ads right, see www.cap.org.uk (Committee of Advertising Practice) and search for 'hypnotherapy.'

You can also take a look at the Hampshire Hypnotherapy website which has been checked out with regards to compliance with advertising standards: www.hampshirehypnotherapist.co.uk

Personal view: sense of community

> Lorraine has built up a community of hypnotherapists among her past students, providing excellent networking opportunities and the chance to continually develop best practice professionally. The ongoing support Lorraine provides is also invaluable, so students do not feel they are left to "get on with it."
> *Jo Fellows, Kallisti Hypnotherapy*

CONCLUSION

Now it is time to think about all you have learned. If you have used this book in conjunction with a practical training course you are well on the way to becoming a hypnotherapist. Just because you have all this knowledge and a diploma, however, it will not bring you clients. You will need to get up and go out there and tell people you are there. Advertise, set up a website, network and give talks. People find hypnosis fascinating, and what we do is so interesting and rewarding.

One of the wonderful things is how in our profession we help people to make positive changes. So whether you decide to develop a business or just practise with your friends and family, I wish you the very best of luck.

If you would like to look at the Hampshire School of Hypnotherapy website, the address is www.hypnoschool.co.uk

We have a Facebook page at www.facebook.com/hampshirehypnotherapy

You can also follow us on Twitter: @hypnohants

We run regular training courses of which you can find full details on the HSH website.

Recommended Reading

Roy Hunter MS, CHt:	The Art of Hypnosis
　　　　　　　　　　　　The Art of Hypnotherapy

Roy Hunter teaches professional hypnosis and was specially selected to carry on the work of the late Charles Tebbetts, a pioneer in hypnotherapy and author of the book Miracles on Demand which is now out of print.

Roger Sleet BA (Hons) Psych, FINT, SQHP: A Guide to Professional Hypnotherapy

Appendix

My Own Experience Of Regression – Never Assume!

When you are regressing people you have to be careful not to make assumptions. I used to be a biscuitaholic (not that I thought so, though I remember one Christmas when Boaster biscuits came on the market I had nine packets bought for me...) My friend Roy joked that he only came to see me for my lovely biscuit tin.

When I was training to be a hypnotherapist my trainer took me into hypnosis and used the IMR. I needed to regress, and this is how it went.

A memory came up of when I was very small and my dad used to take me to work with him. He had his own business as a builder and I loved going on the building sites and seeing the workmen. As a little girl I was very smiley with big brown eyes and my mum used to dress me in lovely little white dresses. How I ever kept them clean I will never know. All the workmen used to make a little fuss of me and I loved it. It may have just been that I was the boss's daughter. On this occasion in my memory I was happily playing on top of a pile of sand and my dad suddenly grabbed me, picked me up, shoved me in the car, handed me a packet of crisps a bottle of Coke and left me there. As an adult I think it was because he needed to tell the workmen off and did not want me to hear. As a little girl I did not know that and felt confused, as I did not understand what I had done wrong!

My trainer asked if this was where it all began. No, was my reply.

Second regression: I went back to nursery school.

I was standing outside and my mum was late as usual. What amazed me was that I felt embarrassed, even at the age of two, because two teachers were there looking at their watches. Anyway, a taxi arrived for me (knowing my mum she was always falling asleep on the sofa and I expect she woke up and looked at the time and phoned our taxi company Maxi Taxi's to pick me up). This happened regularly in my memory. They took me to the taxi office in Havant, in Hampshire, where I used to sit and wait for my mum to come.

My trainer suggested how horrible it must have been sitting in the taxi office with all those men. How wrong could she be? 'Those men' used to be really nice to me and would go across the road to the sweet shop and buy me sweets. I loved it. (I was really angry that my trainer suggested it was horrible – as a hypnotherapist you must be careful, do not assume, just let your client talk. The anger is still there today, even though I understand why. The good thing is it taught me never to assume anything.)

We still weren't where it all began.

Third regression: I went back to being in my gran's house. I was two and I absolutely adored my grandmother. I would follow her to the kitchen. In my regression I could actually feel my nappy moving about as I walked. My grandmother had a butler sink and used to stand there washing up. I would go over and say, 'Granny, what's in the cupboard?' (Knowing full well there were biscuits). She would say, 'I do not know darling, shall we have a look?' She would go over to the cupboard, a great big larder, and open the door and see the biscuits. Then she would say, 'How did they get there! Shall we have one?' And we did.

My trainer asked if this was where it all began? Yes.

What has happened is that when I was a little girl, my subconscious mind knew that when I had those biscuits at my gran's it made me really happy. So when I was unhappy my subconscious mind would produce a behaviour that I would want to eat biscuits as they made me feel happy. As I grew up, I never consciously remembered the events that helped me to have such a wonderful biscuit tin.

The lesson is that when you are using regression, never suggest your client is thinking or feeling anything. Be very, very careful.

There was another incident when a different hypnotherapist was working with me. This time it was about picking on snacks in the evenings. Again, I was about two.

Where are you?
I am under the table.
Are you hiding? (*A leading question. It would have been better to say: 'What are you doing under the table?'*)
No.
What are you doing under the table?
Sitting.
How do you feel?
Okay.
Is anybody there?
Yes.
Who?
My dad and his friends.
How do you feel?

Okay.
What is happening?
They are playing cards.
Why are you hiding under the table?
I am not hiding.
What is happening?

There was a lot of pausing... When you are under hypnosis you do not want to talk, you are processing so much information. You do, however, know what is happening and eventually I chose to tell the therapist.

I said: 'I loved sitting under the table when my dad had his friends round. I was supposed to be in bed, but as long as I was quiet I could stay up. I adored my dad and loved being near him and as I sat next to him under the table he would give me crisps and peanuts.'

The therapist said: 'I want you to see your dad in a circle of light and tell your dad what you need to say.'

I did this.

Then the therapist asked me to cut my dad and all those feelings away. I found this quite stressful as I did not want to cut those feelings away. They were really good feelings, happy feelings. I said this and said I would cut my dad away but not the feelings.

The therapist then did Inner Child. Even though you are under hypnosis you are still able to think, so I did tell the therapist to let me say what I needed to say to the inner child. I did not want the therapist to interpret my inner child.

I was left feeling quite upset about the whole thing. Over the following week I found that my picking at night did not change, but I actually started picking in the day as well. I was fully aware that we did not get to the cause and that we had only just begun. I also feel that the suggestion to cut away good and happy feelings made me want to keep them all the more: hence I started picking in the day.

Meta questioning (how, what, where, when) is so important and simple. It does not lead or suggest. It empowers your client and not you. The regression could have gone like this:

Where are you?
Under the table.
What are you doing under the table?
Sitting.
What is happening?
My dad and friends are playing cards.
How is this connected with your picking in the evening?
I do not know.
How do you think it is connected with your picking in the evening?
Well my dad used to give me crisps and peanuts and I loved it.
Is this where it all began, Yes or No?

At this point I know I would have said No. The therapist would then have continued to regress again.

I do not know at this stage where my subconscious would have taken me. Writing this I am still picking and trying to control my urge to pick during the day.

Regression is a skill that needs to be practised and kept simple. As hypnotherapists it is not our job to analyse the client's problem. Our job is to empower the client and meta questioning is a good way of doing this.

SAMPLE CLIENT CONFIDENTIAL RECORD

NAME: ....

ADDRESS:..
....
....

POST CODE:..

HOME TEL:................................ MOBILE:............................

EMAIL:...

AGE: .... D.O.B: ....

ARE YOU TAKING MEDICATION? IF SO, WHAT? ....
....

WHAT YOU WANT TO ACHIEVE WITH HYPNOTHERAPY:
....
....
....

WHERE DID YOU HEAR ABOUT US:...............................

WOULD YOU LIKE TO RECEIVE INFORMATION ABOUT FUTURE WORKSHOPS AND TIPS   YES/NO

I understand the key to success is *me* and agree to make changes to achieve my goal. I am also aware that hypnotherapy cannot make me do anything I do not wish to do. I appreciate my part in the process and will play the CDs to reinforce the therapy.

Signed:..

Date:..

APPENDIX

SAMPLE MEDICAL MALPRACTICE INSURANCE
Summary of cover

Demands

You are a practitioner/therapist and you have advised us that you require an indemnity to protect you in the event that a claim or allegation is made against you by a patient or third party for malpractice, injury or damage arising from the pursuit of your professional practice.

Needs

We have negotiated a malpractice/public liability policy with Royal and Sun Alliance Insurance PLC. This is arranged on a claims-occurring basis for malpractice/public liability and claims made in respect of legal expenses.

The principal benefits of the cover are detailed as follows:-

- Professional Indemnity – Limit of indemnity £5,000,000 any one event plus unlimited costs in addition. This provides cover for you against claims arising from your neglect error or omission in relation to your professional activities
- Public Liability – Limit of indemnity £5,000,000 any one event plus unlimited costs. This provides cover in respect of legal liability for injury or damage to other parties.
- Products Liability – Limit of indemnity £5,000,000 in any one period of insurance plus unlimited costs. This covers you in respect of injury or damage arising from defects in products sold or supplied by you.
- These covers are extended to include indemnity in respect of libel or slander, breach of confidentiality and Good Samaritan Acts.
- The policy provides cover for teaching provided that you are suitably qualified but there is no cover in respect of the risk of management of the teaching establishment.

- Loss of Documents – there is cover for up to £100,000 in respect of the costs and expenses incurred to restore or replace documents (other than electronic documents)
- Additional therapies may be covered (many without additional cost) provided that you are properly trained and qualified to at least the standards required by the appropriate Professional Bodies or Associations in the chosen therapy.
- Cover applies anywhere in the United Kingdom.

APPENDIX

SAMPLE ACCOUNTS

The Hypnotherapy Practice

Trading and profit and loss account for the year ended 20XX

	£	£
Sales:		15,000
Overhead expenses:		
Rent	2,000	
CPD	200	
Travel & car	1,000	
Stationery & equip incl. web	500	
Membership	240	
Insurance	72	
Repairs & renewals	100	
Advertising	2,000	
Bookkeeping	100	
	6,212	
Profit for the year		**£8,788**